Your Gut Feeling

A Formula for Curing the Incurable

A Remarkable True Story of Healing

Guy Cohen

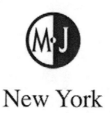

New York

Your Gut Feeling

A Formula for Curing the Incurable

ISBN 978-1-60037-605-4

Library of Congress Control Number: 2009923059

MORGAN · JAMES
THE ENTREPRENEURIAL PUBLISHER

Morgan James Publishing, LLC
1225 Franklin Ave., STE 325
Garden City, NY 11530-1693
Toll Free 800-485-4943
www.MorganJamesPublishing.com

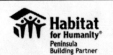

In an effort to support local communities, raise awareness and funds, Morgan James Publishing donates one percent of all book sales for the life of each book to Habitat for Humanity. Get involved today, visit **www.HelpHabitatForHumanity.org**.

Dedication

To Geoffers, because you made all this possible in the first place.
To Dom and Lulu, because you were amazing friends
during those darkest days.
To all the people who have suffered from intestinal problems.
This is for you.

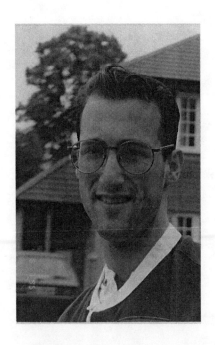 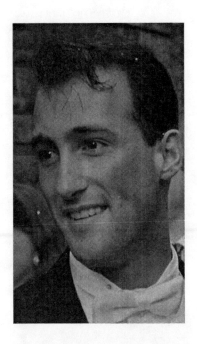

From this—June 1995   To this—August, 1995

Contents

Introduction

I can remember him … vaguely. He was a twenty-three-year-old, normal-looking guy, about five-foot-eleven, with an athletic build, about 168 pounds, and had a cheerful, fun character. An ambitious sort, he was making his way in the real estate business, having completed his undergraduate degree from a reputable university. Destined for success within the industry, in the summer of 1994 the life of this happy-go-lucky young man was taking a dramatic turn … for the worse.

He had noticed a distinct change of mood during the late spring and a constant sense of discomfort in his stomach. This permanent bloated feeling left him irritable and on a short fuse. He was also noticing that he was short of breath and somehow couldn't remember how to breathe comfortably any more. Each breath had to be vigorously sucked in, and yet even that never seemed quite enough.

As spring turned to summer, the bloated feeling continued, and there was the odd bout of diarrhea. Still, he had no serious sense of concern, but he was consciously noticing that his personality was changing. There was this increasingly frequent feeling within his center of a volcano about to erupt and explode out of him. Friends and relatives knew him to be an even-tempered sort, but he was beginning to feel anything but from the inside. His breathing was breathless, and the sensation of wanting to explode in a blaze of fury became almost a daily occurrence. And his stomach was feeling permanently bloated from the moment he rose to the time he went to bed. All this was damaging his relationship. His girlfriend didn't know what was wrong nor what to do about it.

All this was just the prelude to the nightmare that was about to begin. In mid-July 1994 he suffered the first bout of bleeding. Now he was frightened—especially because it came with an acute sense of urgency and the sudden inability to control his movements. Now he definitely had to seek proper help.

As you're reading this story, if you can relate to any of the above physical (or other) warning signs and symptoms described, then keep reading. You understand just how desperate it can be to either have the symptoms of one of the IBD illnesses or watch someone you love suffering from them. As you read on, you'll witness how this man made a 100 percent full recovery. He did it without taking drugs and without resorting to surgery, as was recommended by doctors in both the United Kingdom and the United States only nine months before they pronounced him fully recovered! This book is not a recommendation to do precisely the same but is a true story of how one man decided to build for himself a different reality from the one he was told he'd have to accept. It is also a responsible step-by-step guide on how to build some hope based on a real life story and how you can get started with the right attitude right now.

IBS/ulcerative colitis/Crohn's/diverticulosis is an intensely personal experience, but there are a number of common denominators that you will discover in this book, some of which are sad and others that are just plain funny.

You'll also read how, once he was cured, this man went on to embrace more and more risks and more stress in his life, constantly questioning perceived sources of wisdom before either accepting or rejecting what we all get spoon-fed every day from so-called experts. Never did the condition return, thereby dispelling many of the unquestioned myths that abound about these types of conditions. For this man, he questioned everything he was told that was not constructive to his recovery.

Like I said, I remember this man vaguely. I say only vaguely because he has changed considerably since the time I knew him then. At the time of writing, August 2005, it is now over nine years since he has been completely well. A lot has happened since that time, but the one thing that has been consistent is his overall, general good health. He now runs a successful business built around a product that started as just an idea in his mind. He is now a well-respected pioneer in his field and an international speaker and author, and his clients include some of the largest financial institutions in the world. And he remains completely and consistently healthy.

He has undergone life's ups and downs, including bereavement, heartbreak, work pressures, etc. He was even able to withstand a nasty bout of gastric flu in early 2003, which came and went like it does with any other normal person. It was a short, sharp reminder of how he had existed every day for over a year back in 1994/95. And in making a normal recovery from that gastric flu (one of the main distinctions was a high fever), he realized it was time to share his story with everyone in the world who could identify with the suffering that colitis, Crohn's, or IBS brings with it.

If all this seems slightly incredible to you, it does to me too sometimes, except for the fact that I've known that man all my life— because that man was me.

I am Guy Cohen. I was that man, and I understand every spasm of agony, every sleepless night, every fear, and every tear that goes hand in hand with IBD conditions such as ulcerative colitis or Crohn's.

I am going to share with you all my experiences, including a step-by-step guide of how I made a 100 percent full recovery from the condition. I do not take any medicine. I eat what I like, when I like, and however much I like. I do every activity I want to do, and I take risks that I would never previously have dared to consider. Since I have been well, I have been divorced, broken-hearted, and bereaved. I have taken lots of tests/exams, started businesses, and experienced cloud-nine highs and desperate lows. But the one thing that has remained constant is that I'm fit and healthy, to the point that I can take my good health for granted.

As you're reading this book I want to convey to you a feeling of hope—a feeling that you can have a major input into your own well-being. This is your body. I took responsibility for what was going on in my body. That is not the same as blaming myself. I simply said, "Somehow I must have put it there, and somehow I'm going to have to get rid of it." And I was going to be completely open-minded about the entire process. I didn't care if I had to change. In fact, I welcomed it. If I was the problem, then surely I could do something about me! So many people take issue with this. So many people tell me they're not prepared to change. Why not? If it means improved health leading back to a normal life, why wouldn't you at least consider it? We're not talking changing religions here. We're talking about making small adjustments that can make massive positive differences in your daily life. More on this later.

One important thing to remember is that medical treatment of any form is not a purely scientific process. It's a process of trial and error. Clinical studies are based on double-blind trials involving placebos.

No treatment can be authorized unless a certain statistical target of probability has been reached. With "alternative medicine," the regulatory environment is more of a grey area. As such, medics harbor suspicions, and in some cases rightly so. However, my rule of thumb is simple. If a doctor admits he can't cure you, then why waste time with the doctor? Of course, keep having check-ups to ensure things aren't deteriorating and to keep appraised of the diagnosis itself, but treatment-wise, I knew I'd have to look elsewhere for my answers.

This book is written in three main parts. The first part largely lays out a chronology of my story, what I was thinking, and how I recovered. The second part has more of a documented structure, describing what I did to get better and how it worked. The third section has a bullet-point approach summary of the component parts of my recovery, so you can reference what worked and what didn't work for me. All the sections are important, but this structure means you can always use Part 3 as a reference guide time and time again and chart your own progress. Part 1 is designed to inspire and give hope where it is needed. When I was ill, I scoured the world (the Internet was barely around at the time, so this was a challenge) for people who had made a full recovery from the condition I had (ulcerative colitis), but to no avail. So I took it upon myself to be the first that I'd heard of. Part 2 describes the how and why of my recovery, putting it into replicable structure for you.

When I have to summarize my own recovery I do so in just two parts:

1. Hypnosis and the structure of suggestion
2. The winning attitude

In Part 3 you'll read about the "Rewind Technique". There is no question that had I known about this remarkable application my own recovery would have been dramatically faster.

I know plenty of people with *almost* the right attitude but who haven't applied the structural changes in their thinking patterns required to effect the ultimate progress. I also know people who've gone to hypnotherapy sessions but are averse to being an active part of the change that is required in the healing process.

You must be open to change. And it's really no big deal to change the way you think, especially if it gives you back control over your body and your life! I often hear people say, "I don't want someone controlling my brain." My response is, "Well, either you're not doing a great job of it yourself, so why not have someone else take charge for a while so you can get well or … look at it properly and accept that hypnosis is in fact a *learning* process that enables you to take control of *your own* brain!" That is the truth. And once you're in control, then you can stop arguing with yourself in your own mind, learn how to relax yet be fully active, and enjoy a life without these awful conditions.

When people call me to speak about their problems with UC/ Crohn's/IBS, once they've finished speaking, I gently tell them what's going on in their minds and how they think. They're always astonished. They often start to weep because they know I understand what they're going through. Sometimes they become angry because they find it intrusive, and occasionally they'll get offended because instinctively I'll know precisely what's going on in their mind—and I always tell them! None of this is magic, but believe me, it can seem like it. Even I sometimes surprise myself with it, because it feels like a special power, but it's not. It all comes about through an intense understanding I have of these conditions because of my own intense and personal experiences. All I ask you to do here is be open-minded and be honest. Be honest with yourself.

When I was ill, I was so desperate, I would have done *anything* to get well again. I want you to ask yourself how desperate you are to get well again and put all this behind you for good. I'm going to keep asking you this as we go along in this book. I didn't want merely an improvement. I wanted to be right back to normal, for good. That was my attitude, and nothing was going to stop me pursuing it. If, by reading my story, you can replicate elements of my attitude, then you'll be well on your way. I even stopped speaking with people who didn't believe in me. This meant that I didn't speak with many people, because the perceived wisdom is that it's not possible. But it is possible, because I did it and it's documented. Now it's your turn to read how I did it and what steps you can take to copy what I did.

How to Use This Book

If you want to make the most of this book, you'll want to download the digital audio relaxation recordings that are on the website www. yourgutfeeling.com. The recordings cost less than a single session with a therapist, and you can use them whenever you feel the need for the rest of your life. The effects will be noticeable.

The first track is the original digital copy of Geoffrey Glassborow's hypnotherapeutic induction that is specific to IBD. This is the very recording I took with me to Portland, Oregon, when I was getting married in 1995. I was away from home for almost six weeks and unable to see Geoffrey, so listening to this was the next best thing. By listening to the recording every day, I made astonishing progress and was able to fully enjoy my wedding and honeymoon. In Part 1 below, you'll see the before and after photos of me from June 1995 to August 1995. My transformation owes much to this recording. The second track is another hypnotic recording, this time with accompanying alpha wave frequency music.

You'll also want to interact with the Rewind Technique recording, which you can also download from www.yourgutfeeling.com.

To get the most from this course, you should read this book, listen to your favored track reasonably frequently, and fully participate in the Rewind Technique. You may wish to start by listening to your preferred track (or both) several times a week, and then as you notice an improvement, you can gradually ease off.

As with all things in life, I value the power of encouragement and inspiration. That's what works for me. I believe that anyone can do what I did, provided they have the right information and the right attitude. All the information I know is contained here. The attitude has to come from within, though it's also my job to inspire you to new heights. I hope by reading my story you'll start to feel that tingle of excitement that you can do it too. You can look forward to a healthy future and a life of freedom. You can copy the things I did, and you can get the results you crave. The healthy state is the natural state, and you deserve to be well. So let's get to work!

Guy Cohen

What Is IBD?

Inflammatory Bowel Disorder (IBD) spans a range of evils, including ulcerative colitis, diverticulosis, and Crohn's disease. On a lesser level, we can include Irritable Bowel Syndrome (IBS), which is a less serious condition, yet with similar symptoms of extraordinary discomfort.

For the purposes of this book, we're making the following distinctions:

- What I had was ulcerative colitis.
- We'll work with my collective definition of IBD to include IBS, ulcerative colitis, and Crohn's disease. They are effectively of the same family. If your problem is IBS, then your symptoms aren't quite as severe as with Crohn's or colitis.
- In my experience, and for the practical purposes of this course, there are crucial common denominators between these different conditions. Crucially, these common denominators are particularly pertinent for the way in which we are going to attack the particular condition in hand.

So, we start with the premise that IBS, ulcerative colitis, and Crohn's disease are part of the same family of inflammatory bowel disorders, though with different degrees of severity. Diverticulosis presents itself slightly differently in a physical sense, however, typically not in an emotional sense, so we include it in our definitions.

For clinically official and orthodox definitions, please go to the Appendix. I would emphasize that this course is not about definitions. It's about getting better and better until the condition isn't there any more. That's why we put things like definitions in the back.

Parts of this book were not easy for me to write. I specifically mean the parts that described the illness itself and how it affected me at the time. To do justice to my story, it involved delving back into the archives of my memory, recalling what had happened. This was a chapter of my life that I had long consigned to the past. I didn't really want to associate with the person who had gone through what I went through. These things are very personal, and we all have our different ways of handling things. However, now that it's done, and you're about to read all about it, it feels good, particularly because it's where it belongs … in the past.

PART ONE—My Story

May 1994—Storm Clouds Gathering

Was I healthy before I got ulcerative colitis in the summer of 1994? You bet I was—and active too. I was not a health freak, just a normal athletic kind of guy. I'd never been overweight and had always been into participative sports, and there was absolutely no indication of any troubles ahead.

So let's go back to May 1994, when I had a completely healthy disposition. Looking back with hindsight, the process started slowly. It started with a bloated sensation in my abdomen. It was a busy time socially, and there were lots of meals out, parties, and long spring evenings. I put the bloated feeling down to simple over-indulgence and assumed it would go away the next day. But it didn't go away, so I assumed it would go the next day. But it still didn't go away. If anything, it just got worse. June continued in much the same way as May. I still wasn't overly worried, just uncomfortable, so I just carried on as normal.

One thing that was noticeably different was my mood. I've always been pretty even-tempered. But from that May in 1994, I seemed to have developed an unusually short fuse. My breathing was tense, shallow, and breathless, and I was aware of the fact that I could hardly ever yawn, as I simply couldn't get the breath in. I also noticed that I was becoming highly agitated in my mind. I was constantly having conflicts with people in my mind. During one lunch break at work, I even remember looking forward to having a walk in the park and having this argument with someone in my mind! Looking back, these were the warning signs that I simply didn't understand without the benefit of hindsight.

July 1994—The Nightmare Begins

But in July things changed. The symptoms took a serious turn for the worse. I was now experiencing serious urgency and was struggling not to get "caught short" several times a day. The first time was at work where I had to run out of a meeting twice in fifteen minutes. Finally, one day I noticed the bleeding … lots of it. I remember a wave of silent panic engulfing me when I first saw it. I was scared. I didn't want to even contemplate what could be going on. All I knew was that I had to tell my girlfriend, Kelly, and see a doctor as soon as possible. Before seeing my physician, we speculated that perhaps it could be hemorrhoids (piles). If only—because that would then be funny! But something was telling me that it was not going to be quite so simple.

An appointment with a specialist was confirmed for the following week, but in the meantime, Kelly and I were going to Paris for a romantic weekend. It was my first time to see Paris, and what should have been a fun weekend was partially clouded by the fact that I had to be near a men's room for fear of having an accident. By this time my GP had confirmed that what I had was definitely not piles but something he referred to as "colitis." At this stage he described it as a nuisance and said not to worry too much, the specialist gastroenterologist would do a thorough examination. That was something to look forward to! The reality was that I was anxious to get a proper diagnosis ... and then treatment.

The day after returning home, I had the appointment with the specialist. He was the father of an acquaintance from my old school, so it wasn't particularly dignified when he asked me to undress and lie on my left hand side in preparation for the dreaded "up-periscope"!

After he'd taken the biopsies and had a good look around, the doctor then explained it would take a few days to get the results and for him to tell me his diagnosis. I also had to make another appointment for an X-ray, to be preceded by a barium enema. These examinations are thoroughly unpleasant and also involve the various medical instruments blowing air up the rectum, which is uncomfortable to say the least. The doctor's instinct was pointing towards Crohn's disease, but he also thought it could be colitis. When the test results came back a few days later, he still couldn't make his mind up. Not really understanding the implications, I didn't like this lack of a definitive diagnosis. It just made me more concerned that perhaps he was hiding something from me. Ulcerative colitis was the more likely of the two, but he wasn't going to rule out Crohn's. In the meantime I was prescribed sulphur drugs (sulphazalazine) and corticosteroids (prednisolone or prednisone) to calm everything down. I assumed this would be a course that would last a couple of months and then everything would be back to normal.

As the weeks went by, the drugs seemed to be masking the urgency, but the bleeding was getting worse. This didn't make me feel particularly confident about the drugs I was taking, and in the meantime, the dosages were being increased.

But it wasn't until December of 1994, over four months after the non-diagnosis and with the symptoms getting worse and worse, that I thought to ask the specialist the very simple question: "When am I going to get well from this?"

His answer was vague. He spoke of "dousing the flames" but didn't give me a definitive answer. And I didn't ask for one. By now I was so frightened that I really didn't want to encourage any answers I didn't want to hear. Night time was especially lonely. Although I was with my partner every night, there was no way she could understand the mental torment that was going on with this. From the time the bleeding started, for over a year I never had one full night's sleep, either because of the symptoms or because of the fear.

December 1994—The Realization

For Christmas 1994, I went to Kelly's parents' in Portland, Oregon. As my future in-laws, they were very concerned about me and displayed real kindness that I will always remember. They insisted that I go to see their gastroenterologist in Portland. It was December 30, 1994, and I was up for anything in order to be cured. They gave me such confidence in their specialist that I already had a good feeling about the appointment. Maybe he would find something different to what they were saying in the United Kingdom, and then I'd be well very soon. As the consultation loomed, I had a real sense of optimism.

The consultation was professional enough. Without going into sordid detail, I was led by the nurses and prepared for the "up-periscope," this one involving a meter-long hose with a camera and instruments for the biopsies. There was no sedative (there was in the United Kingdom for this particular joyous experience), and I was able to watch the entire movie of my bowels live in glorious Technicolor.

Afterward it was time to get dressed and have the consultation. I was told that I did have ulcerative colitis and that I should use sulphazalazine enemas as opposed to the tablets. So, right there and then, I bought enough for three months on the spot!

As I prepared to leave, I turned to the doctor, now full of optimism. I assumed that the enemas would be more effective and would therefore cure me. I asked, "So, when am I going to get better?"

"What do you mean, better?" the doctor replied. I didn't like the sound of his tone, and for the first time it dawned on me that we weren't talking the same language,

"Well, completely cured ..." I proffered tentatively. I didn't know that this was the moment at which point my entire destiny was about to change.

The doctor's response to my question shocked me. I couldn't believe anyone could be so callous and insensitive, particularly a doctor recommended by my "in-laws." His response was to laugh out loud in my face, cheerfully telling me that I'd never be well and that I'd simply have to live with the problem for the rest of my life. My reaction was one of pure fury. I went berserk, exploding with a tirade of four letter profanities directed straight at him! Significantly, I also swore I *would* get well and that I'd make sure he'd eat his words one day.

As I was frog marched out of the hospital, a big bag of enemas on both my arms, I had become transformed. Suddenly I knew my fate was going to be decided not by any doctor but by me. How dare he say I couldn't get well? I'd show him ... and show everyone else who didn't believe I could do it. All of my fury was now being channeled positively into my imagination. Even at that time I was visualizing my recovery.

This type of reaction to what the doctor had so callously told me is known as a polarity response. Polarity responders, like me, will do the precise opposite of what they're told is possible. In this case, I was told it was impossible for me to get back to full fitness. My mission was set firm from that moment on. And now I knew where *not* to go in order to achieve my goal. Doctors!

In the New Year of 1994/95, I had no idea what to expect. All I knew was that I was preoccupied, with only one thing on my mind. It was becoming clear to me that in order to achieve the impossible, I was going to have to play a major role in my own recovery. As I took the flight back home to London, I started to formulate my plan. One thing at the back of my mind was that in that November 1994, I had attended a self-improvement workshop where I'd walked over hot coals. I pieced together the logic that if I could get my body to walk over 1000-degree Fahrenheit burning coals, then surely I could get it to do something else, like restore myself back to full health. If nothing else, I was determined to use the fire-walk as a metaphor for my own recovery. It gave me hope, and that's about all I had.

Back home, my first course of action was to conduct as much research as possible. In 1995, the Internet was something for the future, and there was very little information available immediately to hand. The only real sources were medical journals (no use to me by now), health food shops (of which there weren't many because this was before the health food craze of the early 2000s,) and hearsay. Research was clearly going to have to be an ongoing project.

My first major decision was what to do about the drugs I'd been taking. Still in a haze of emotion, I was so disillusioned with the medical profession that I simply flushed them all down the toilet. Tablets, enemas, and suppositories, you name them, they all went! Was this a smart thing to do? Probably not, but I was a man on a mission now. I was going to do this my way, and I didn't want anything to mask the symptoms. I had made the decision that only a complete recovery back to normal was going to be acceptable to me.

January 1995—A Spiral of Decline

The result of trashing all the drugs meant that I could now feel every spasm of agony, and the urgency came back to unprecedented levels. I was still having check-ups with my specialist in London but was taking no medicines from him. He was simply there now to see that the diagnosis was the same.

I was now fully committed to the alternative medicine route. My first port of call was to a homeopath at the Hale Clinic in London. As I was about to discover over the next six months, all of the alternative practitioners I met were 100 percent confident that they would cure me. Wanting to believe everything positive I heard, I flung myself into every type of treatment with complete conviction. I even started celebrating the fact that I would indeed make a full recovery one day and would visualize it in great detail. I didn't know at the time just how important these daydreams could be.

The homeopath suggested that I had the *Helicobacter pylori* bacteria and that was causing the ulcerative colitis. He immediately put me on a special diet involving no wheat and put me on a course of natural homeopathic antibiotics to eliminate the bug. I also had to provide a stool sample so they could confirm the bug was there. It is well documented that peptic ulcers can be caused by helicobacter pylori, and the thinking here was that the bacteria must also be causing the ulceration and inflammation in my colon. It actually seemed logical to me, and I went into the treatment with the attitude that I'd soon be back to normal.

Unfortunately, there was one major snag with this treatment. The tests came back and showed there was no *Helicobacter pylori* present at all. This was a major blow. Over the period of several weeks, my hopes with the homeopath had been completely shattered. My confidence had taken a beating, and almost immediately I noticed my symptoms were getting worse. I was now deteriorating to the point that I needed to go to the toilet over ten times per day, each time with about a one-minute warning coming, with severe pain in the rectum. The bleeding was ever-present. How I prayed for the day that would stop—and I wasn't even religious!

February 1995—The Quest for a Cure

And so began my long search for a cure. Anything would do. I didn't care what it would take, I would do anything. I'd believe the moon was made of cheese if it meant I could be better again. I hated what had now become a prison sentence. I was struggling to have a social life because I was not only being careful about what I ate but the increasing urgency was also having a serious impact on my ability to get out and about. I was, however, determined to press on and live as normal a life as possible. I didn't want what was fast becoming a disability to affect my life any more than it already was. The truth was, though, that the colitis was dominating my life. But I was determined to dominate the colitis.

I was continuing my research on a number of fronts. On one level I was having massage and reflexology therapy from a lady who claimed to have been cured from colitis, and on another I had discovered a Chinese herbal doctor who seemed to know what he was doing.

Before we recount the Chinese herbal medicine in more depth, it's worth talking about the reflexologist. As she was tending to my feet, she told me very firmly that my breathing was too shallow and that I needed to learn how to breathe. She also told me that it was only after she had left her husband, changed her life, and learned to breathe that her condition had improved and cleared up. My overwhelming feeling was that she was exaggerating things and that she simply couldn't have had what I was suffering from. It didn't seem feasible that breathing techniques and a change in one's personal circumstances could possibly be a cure for colitis. I knew she was being genuine and not trying to rip me off. But I also considered her to be a quack. With hindsight, although she wasn't the one to get me well, I have considerably more respect for her views now, thirteen years later. The problem at the time was that I didn't have any faith in her, and I wasn't getting any results from her treatments, pleasant though they were.

At this time, the symptoms were spiraling out of control. I was having to go to the toilet at totally unpredictable times. I was in complete agony, the warning time was shortening, and I was still bleeding every time. The gastroenterologist was still doing his "up-periscope" on me every three weeks. In March 1995, he suggested surgery as my best course of action. I asked if surgery would cure me. He said it wouldn't necessarily be a cure, and then added, almost as an aside, that it would mean a colostomy bag too. I told him to fuck off!

The Chinese herbal treatment involved a number of components. The main part was the medicine itself, which was absolutely disgusting. If you've ever tried it, you'll know what I mean. I had to boil up bits of tree bark and other weird shrubbery in water and then drink the tea twice a day, every day. I can only wince at the memory of it! But if it was going to make me better, then I was going to do it—anything it took. More pleasantly, on each visit to the Chinese doctor, he would administer some acupuncture, which sent me to sleep every time, and burn incense inside a box he'd put on my stomach. This too was very nice but none too effective.

April–May 1995—My Nadir

By April 1995, I was just about reaching my nadir. I counted at one point that I was going to the toilet over thirty times a day. Even passing wind was a trauma of excruciating pain and always involved passing blood. Effectively, I was incontinent, and there were occasions even during meetings at work where I was clenching for my life before running out as discretely as possible. And sometimes I didn't make it. I was completely stripped of my dignity. Half my life seemed to be spent sitting on the toilet in spasms of agony. Nothing seemed to be having any positive effect on me. No treatment seemed to be working. The gastroenterologist told me that in a range of one to ten, with ten being bad, my condition was now measured at eight out of ten. Again, he suggested alternatives. Again I told him to go away, as I had done before! I was still searching. I still believed I could find a way to get better. I didn't care how long it was going to take (well, actually I did!), but I was never going to give up on this. I was never going to give up on myself. Somehow I'd find a way.

It was around Easter in 1995 that I discovered a woman who owned a health food shop near where I was living in London. When I met her, I was in a state. She told me she could help. In fairness, they all did. But this woman had serious conviction about her abilities as a naturopath, and I latched onto her self-belief. We made an appointment, and yet again I was filled with feelings of great hope and anticipation.

The consultation was professional and at the end she gave me her assessment. She could get me completely well in a matter of weeks provided I follow her instructions to the absolute letter. Those instructions mainly consisted of the most rigid diet I have ever seen. Remember that at this stage I was still sticking to the diet given to me by the homeopath back in January. I'd only lost about eight pounds in weight and was around 160 pounds. Just to give you an idea, this woman's diet consisted of the following:

Breakfast:	Homemade oat bread (oats mixed with water, then baked in the oven) with plain, unsalted churned butter.
Lunch:	Plain grilled organic chicken with raw vegetables, including broccoli, carrots, and cucumber.
Dinner:	A boiled onion with boiled greens (I blended this into a soup, which wasn't too bad) and a baked potato with plain, unsalted churned butter.

Nothing else was permitted. I could eat as much of the above as I wanted, but everything had to be homemade and freshly prepared. I followed this diet to the letter. And I lost a lot of weight over the next two months.

Almost two months into this particular course of treatment, in May 1995, I even spent a week under constant supervision by the naturopath woman. I was forbidden to watch TV and was only allowed to drink the fresh vegetable juices she prepared in the juicer and take walks in the countryside. She even had me insert raw fresh garlic … from behind, if you get my meaning! I really can't recommend it. It seriously stings—and didn't do any good either!

When I came back from this adventure, my weight was at its lowest, I had lost another thirty pounds and was weighing in at about 130 lbs. People who got to see me privately whispered among each other how long I'd got and thought I was dying. I wasn't—but I wasn't exactly living either. You can see the pictures later in this chapter. The symptoms were still horrific, and I was still frightened. I wasn't getting any better, but crucially, I wasn't getting any worse either. Mind you, at eight out of ten, there wasn't much worse I could get.

At this stage, it's worth mentioning my personal relationships with family, friends, and my fiancée at the time. Most friends simply didn't know what to do and where to put themselves. There were a few wonderful exceptions. One group of friends even came up with a new nickname for me … Guy Colon! As such, Kelly and I were named "the Colons"! I don't blame the other friends who effectively stayed away. It must have been scary for them to watch me wasting away like that. I wasn't able to be sociable at all, and I had by now developed an obsession with getting back to full health. Anyone who didn't believe I could get better wasn't welcome to communicate with me. Not many people believed I could get better, so I simply didn't speak with many people.

My family was the same. They had asked around their doctor friends and had been told emphatically that I was wasting my time trying to find a cure. They relayed this to me, and I ignored them too. You just cannot take away someone's hope or spirit, and I refused to listen to anything that threatened my convictions of hope. Kelly was fantastic when it came to preparing meals from the absurdly limited ingredients that were permitted, but understandably, she struggled emotionally with all this. Since that pivotal doctor's appointment in Portland, all my energy was now focused on doing the impossible. I wasn't prepared to live my life as a prison sentence, not when I was only twenty-four. What kind of husband could I be anyway if I was stuck on the toilet in agony all the time? My logic was that I simply had no choice but to fight and somehow find a solution.

Slowly but surely I began to realize that this naturopath woman was more of a dangerous, mad eccentric than savior for me, and I started looking at other methods again. One of the things that bothered me about her was that she was very controlling. It was her way or the highway. I started to remember the fire walk back in November, and how I could use that experience to make me better. I'd always been fascinated by hypnosis and the power of the mind. For many years we'd had a family friend called Geoffrey who had a fearsome reputation as a hypnotherapist. After years of suffering with depression, my mother had seen this man just a few times and was cured. But I had a problem with him. The problem was that I didn't want to hear the word no from anyone, and in particular I didn't want to hear it from *him*. So I didn't contact him.

Instead I went to other people. Spiritualists, healers, you name it, I went there! I had my auras cleaned, my spirit cleansed, my karma balanced. Nothing worked. I wasn't getting any worse (I was still an eight out of ten), but I wasn't getting any better. Eventually I did go to a hypnotherapist. As the appointment unfolded, she did put me into a trance and I did feel relaxed, but there were a couple of major issues. First, she had never treated my condition before, and second, it was clear that she was very inexperienced, since she was reading out the induction. I needed someone a lot more experienced than her. I needed someone who'd seen it all, someone I could not only trust but whom I could also respect and have faith in. I only knew of one such person, and frightening though it was, I finally plucked up the courage to pick up the phone and dial Geoffrey's number.

June 1995—The Turning Point

Of course he knew who I was and greeted me like an old friend. We'd only met once before at a party, and he was like your favorite, lively grandfather. He was already seventy-three years old at the time, and it was clear that he was a man with enormous life experience as well as professional experience. Our phone conversation was direct, yet very warm. Yes, he'd seen this (colitis) before, yes, he'd treated it successfully, and yes, he was confident he could help. First he wanted to see me so we could chat through it. As we made the appointment, I was welling up with emotion and submerged with waves of goose-bumps going up and down my spine. Already this was feeling very different than all that had gone on before.

I implicitly trusted Geoffrey, and my biggest fear (of him saying no) hadn't materialized. Unlike all the other people I'd seen, I knew for sure that Geoffrey would never give me hope based on false pretenses.

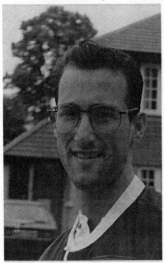

This is what I looked like when I went for that first appointment with Geoffrey in June 1995. I was still seeing the eccentric naturopath woman, and even she was alarmed about my weight loss. I'd always been a well-built guy, and now I was reduced to skin and bone. Accordingly, I was now "permitted" to eat an organic egg every day plus a fillet steak. Can you imagine how nice that felt after being confined to that diet for the previous two months? And I had never once cheated on that diet either, so this felt like luxury.

Most people who saw me at the time were pretty shocked, especially if they'd known me in years gone by. There were worse pictures than this, but at the time I threw them all away, not knowing that one day I would be writing a book about the experience. And while on that subject, it's worth noting that now, as an experienced author, this has not been an easy book to write. As I alluded to in the introduction, I barely associate with the person I was at the time simply because the memories are so harrowing. This is one of the reasons I don't go into too much detail about the suffering and indignity of what I went through.

June 1995—Learning How to Think

So off I went for my first appointment with Geoffrey. I immediately felt at ease when I met this lively grandfatherly figure with his dog by his side at his country practice. I sat on the recliner chair, and we started to chat. He told me that at the end of our chat he would tell me how he could help. He asked me what I was looking to achieve from this, and I made it very clear I was only interested in a complete cure and making the illness part of my past.

I then went into great detail about my symptoms and how I wanted to get better. I even went into detail about how I wanted to feel when I did get better! It was at this point that the learning process, and the magic, started.

Geoffrey said, "Well, how about we make your goal to be totally fit?"

I said, "Yes, but I want to go to the toilet no more than three times a day, and I don't want there to be any urgency, and I don't want there to be any bleeding, and I don't want there to be any pain ..."

Geoffrey replied, "So how about we just say you'll be totally fit? You see, if you're totally fit, you wouldn't have any of those symptoms anyway, would you?"

This was the first of many salient lessons I started to learn and appreciate from Geoffrey. If I simply imagined myself vibrant, fit, and well, that would embrace all the things I wanted to achieve. I didn't need to think about the details of the recovery. If I was fit, then the illness simply wouldn't be there anyway. Already I was beginning to see what was happening here. Geoffrey was essentially teaching me how to think, which is something we don't get taught at school. Bad thinking can lead to bad health. Simple ... and true. In my case, chronically so.

The first session continued, and for the last twenty minutes Geoffrey went through his hypnotic induction and specific words for my particular case. Professionally speaking, Geoffrey is a psychotherapist who uses hypnotherapy as a tool. This is significant, because a deep knowledge of psychology and philosophy are essential ingredients. Combined with hypnosis, this enables Geoffrey to work some serious magic. In my mind at the time, I was seeing a hypnotist! But the results Geoffrey is able to achieve, even now at eighty-six years old in his country practice, owe much to his multidisciplinary professional background as well as a wisdom earned over many years and countless experiences.

Before the hypnosis began, I asked Geoffrey what he thought of my particular case. His reply was emphatic. "We'll get you right. That I am very confident about."

I asked, "How right?"

"Totally fit," he replied. "We'll make this a thing of the past."

Already I was feeling energized by his confidence.

I asked him how long it would take for me to get completely well again. In return, he asked me how long I thought would be reasonable. He then went on. "Well, obviously a day would be too short for a recovery from this, but I think a year would be too long." And so we went back and forth, "negotiating" on how long we thought this should take. And we settled on six months, just in time for Christmas and New Year.

I was due to get married in August, so we also aimed for a marked improvement by that time. It was at this point that Geoffrey revealed another invaluable insight.

He explained that nothing in life could ever be represented purely by a straight, uninterrupted line. In other words, any line on a graph always has retracements. "Your recovery will be the same. You'll get a surge of improvement and then nothing for a little while before it starts to improve again. But provided the trend is always upward, you'll get there. You'll get the complete recovery you're looking for. What we're going to do is to ensure that the trend is in the right direction from now on."

It all sounded so logical. It was pure common sense. How the use of words was going to effect this change was another matter, but I now knew for sure that this man knew exactly what he was doing.

"Now, let's get to work," he said.

I didn't go to sleep at all during that hypnosis. I was awake, albeit very relaxed, during the entire thing, but I absolutely knew I was in the presence of a master here. His experience was so obvious that I felt assured from the start. It didn't matter that I didn't sleep, because you don't need to be sleeping for the positive hypnotic suggestions to sink in. I had a sense that something was already changing, though I wasn't quite sure what or how.

There was only one small snag. Because I was due to go to Oregon for my wedding, it meant we were only able to have a few sessions before my travels. So we had a second session only a few days after the first. There was no doubt that something was changing inside me, but I couldn't put a finger on it. Physically there was no change, but mentally some very powerful shifts were occurring.

By the time I'd had the first session with Geoffrey I'd already given up my job in order to concentrate on getting well again. This was a huge risk but one I felt had to be taken. What use was I to anyone in my ill state anyway? One of my (by now former) work colleagues had invited me and Kelly to his engagement party almost two hundred miles away the weekend after my second session with Geoffrey. Typically at that time I'd have declined the invitation, but we left it provisionally open, and after that second session, I told Kelly I thought we should go.

Even she was noticing a slight change in me. I was inwardly becoming more relaxed and this was already translating to my outward behavior. Kelly asked me what I'd do about food, since at that time we were still preparing everything strictly in accordance with that appalling diet. I said we'd prepare enough for twenty-four hours and that I simply wouldn't eat anything at the party.

So, we made the journey up north and attended. About one hour into the party I was looking at the food on offer—which looked very tempting as usual—but now I was looking at the food in a totally different way. I remember looking at all the crudités and thinking to myself, *I don't think you're the problem.* This was a massive mind shift. Remember, for over six months now I had been on one strict dietary regime or another, and for the past two months I'd been in a dietary straightjacket. I kept eyeing up the food and gingerly approached the counter and popped one of the luxurious morsels in my mouth. Kelly suddenly rushed up to me. "What are you doing?" she cried as I was chewing away.

"It's OK," I replied, "I don't think it'll be a problem."

"Jeez, there really is something going on with you!"

And so there was. Over the next twenty four hours there was no change whatsoever in my physical state, thereby proving to me that in my particular case food was not the problem. That didn't mean that I was going to go wild or anything, but it meant that I could slowly but surely ease myself back to a normal diet. As my confidence started to grow, this took a few months, but the straightjacket was off, and I could now stop wasting my time on things that weren't working.

Crucially, Geoffrey had not mentioned one thing about food, neither in the hypnosis nor in our conversations, other than to say that of course one day I'd eat normally again. Little did I know that meant almost right away! But as you'll hear for yourself, he didn't mention food within the hypnosis itself. Somehow my subconscious mind was beginning to work out where I needed to concentrate my energies in order for me to get well again. Physically I felt no real difference immediately after those first two sessions. However, emotionally and psychologically the engagement party proved to be an enormous leap for me, and within a few days I was noticing a distinct improvement physically too. This was after just two sessions with Geoffrey.

At this point I had another appointment with the gastroenterologist. I was intrigued to hear what he had to say after the up-periscope. My confidence was building, and I even began joking with him, asking him whether he ever told his wife what he did during the day! Kelly sat behind the screen playfully admonishing me as my lavatorial sense of humor started to return. After the gloves were off, I asked the doctor what he thought and he said, "Well, there's a definite improvement." I asked him what mark out of ten I had now, and he replied about a six. This was a real improvement from the eight he'd given me before (remember, ten was bad). And this again was after just two sessions with Geoffrey. Now I was convinced as to the root cause of the condition, and I asked the doctor if he would let me have just a couple of tranquilizers for the next two months that I was going to be away. He acceded to my request, knowing that I was averse to taking any medicine from him anyway! He explained that some tranquilizers can be addictive. I replied that they should be the lowest possible dose and I'd only use them in the event of a real emergency to take the edge off any serious anxiety. In the next two months I only took two halves of one pill!

I had one more appointment with Geoffrey before going off to get married in Oregon. During this session, Geoffrey recorded the hypnosis so I could listen to it whenever I wanted while I was away. When you download the recordings from www.yourgutfeeling.com, this is the first one. I listened to it almost every day, and my health continued to improve while I was away. This was almost unimaginable just a few weeks before. After just three sessions, my entire thinking habits were in the process of changing. I was noticing things about the way I had been thinking and how self-destructive those habits had been. I started to notice how my body was changing. I was still nowhere near well, but the trend had most definitely changed, and the spiral of decline had been arrested. I was making noticeable changes internally that filled me with belief and hope. I knew I was on my way back, and our negotiated target of six months was looking realistic.

August 1995—Wedding Bells

Although the marriage didn't ultimately last more than a few years, the wedding itself and honeymoon were fun and memorable. That's not to say they were without the odd emotional up-and-down, but by and large, it was a happy time made better by the fact that I was continuing to make giant strides health-wise.

My new in-laws were fantastic. On this visit, they introduced me to their own naturopath, and although I was happy with the progress I was making with Geoffrey, I was equally happy to supplement it with herbal remedies if appropriate. This time the naturopath was very sweet and helpful. She was an agent for Nature's Sunshine herbal products and soon had me on a range of natural gelatine capsules ranging from capsicum to slippery elm bark! There were other potions I adopted with her, and none of them did any harm. I'm not sure any of them did any good either, but they were natural, low-hassle, and I thought, *Why not?* Now that I'd canned the strict regimental diets, I still wanted to do something physically to help myself, even if it was the psychological side that was actually working.

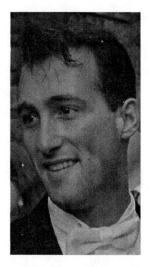

Only about seven weeks after that first photo, this is what I looked like. By now I had regained about twenty pounds in weight (about half of what I had lost), and I was a different person. I still had a fair way to go to make a full recovery, but I was now on the upward curve. The momentum was with me, and my confidence was growing. And I was able to enjoy my time away from home too. This would have been unthinkable only weeks before.

October 1995—Stalling and Retracements

By October I was a different person. I was still not completely well, but what a difference from March when I was being told to have surgery. The bleeding was settling down. Sometimes there was none at all and the pan wasn't red when I'd finished. The frequency was well below ten times per day—more around five to seven—and the urgency and pain were far less than before. The gastroenterologist now had me at just four out of ten. There was only one problem. I seemed to be stuck at that level for several weeks. Geoffrey had explained to me from the outset that there would be periods during the recovery that would seem a bit frustrating and where little progress would be in evidence. His wisdom and experience was crucial here, because without it I may have done something silly like pursue something else. I'd already enjoyed such monumental results, and I was getting impatient to finish the job off.

I started looking at alternatives to hypnosis while still keeping up with Geoffrey's treatments. I searched high and low and found a highly reputable practitioner in New York. We scheduled a phone call, and I explained the entire situation, even quoting Geoffrey in terms of anticipating this lull period where the improvement appeared to be in suspense. After an hour's conversation, the consultant told me to stick to what I was doing, as he not only couldn't think of anything better, but also had learned a lot himself purely in the course of our conversation! Not that I should have needed it, but this gave me another huge boost to know that someone of good repute was endorsing what I was doing. He was turning down the opportunity to make decent money from me and confirmed that I was definitely on the right track, in his professional opinion. I remember that night vividly, and I celebrated the knowledge that I'd soon be completely well again by doing one of the most uncoordinated dance routines ever performed on this planet before my wife got back home!

I spoke earlier about my changing thinking habits. It was around this time that I started to consciously realize that my thinking habits had really changed and that things didn't bother me in the same way as they always had before. I noticed that I wasn't arguing internally with myself any more. In fact, every time I was tempted to have an imaginary argument with a friend or relative in my mind, I'd cut it short by asking myself rhetorical questions. Such as, *Guy, why are you doing this? What possible good is this doing you? Are you getting anything constructive from this?* And then I'd end up laughing to myself about it. Fancy that. Spending my spare time arguing with myself! How ridiculous was that! Yet it had been the way I'd thought since I was a young teenager.

Years later when I was on a Richard Bandler course, he started talking about this very phenomenon, and once again I smiled to myself in the knowledge that I knew exactly what he was talking about. It gave me the feeling that although I had already eliminated those destructive thinking habits a while back, at least I knew I had not been alone! Richard's technique for putting a stop to those self-flagellating internal arguments was slightly different than mine. Whereas I had used the rhetorical questions technique to tease myself into better habits, he advocated the "shut the fuck up" technique where you notice the self-arguments and then tell yourself to "shut the fuck up" repeatedly!

Another major aspect that I was now consciously aware of was my breathing. It's incredible how powerful this is. I have several friends who've had abdominal issues, and I've taught them how to breathe. Literally in minutes they're feeling more comfortable. Be more consciously aware of your breathing. It's crucial to your overall good health. Most people breathe too shallowly; it's a commonly known fact. Try slowing your breathing down, both in and out. Unfocus your eyes by gently crossing them and take a long, slow, deep breath. Make sure you're sitting at the time! There are a few other things that you should try that we'll look at in more detail in the next section.

Remember too about Geoffrey's trendlines on a graph. In life, nothing ever occurs in a straight line. The stock markets, your favorite sports teams, your own life patterns, your health, you name it—life consists of ebbs and flows. In terms of your own health, provided the trend is going in the right direction, you'll get where you want to be. See the graph below. It depicts this perfectly. There are several ups and downs, but the overall trend is up. In my recovery there weren't so many downs per se, but there were a few weeks where the graph went sideways. That's totally natural and was evidently so in the context of my overall recovery.

Upward-Trending "Recovery" Graph

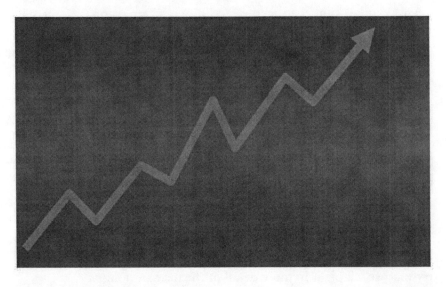

November–December 1995—
In the Final Straight

Once my belief was restored, it wasn't long before I started noticing another real surge of improvement. The bleeding was getting less and less, and in November the specialist had me marked down to a two out of ten. He said, "I don't know how you're doing it, but I guess you're some sort of statistical phenomenon." I turned to him, somewhat mystified, and said, "You know exactly how I'm doing it."

I told him about every alternative therapy I was pursuing so he would be in the picture. What annoyed me was that he was putting this down to luck. Yet this was scientific. I was at my absolute worst when I met Geoffrey, and since the treatments had begun, I was making giant strides of improvement. And this doctor, whose job was supposed to be to help people, was blatantly ignoring something right in front of his very eyes. He was a first-hand witness to this entire process and had noted improvements since the summer. He knew I wasn't doing anything else, I was taking no drugs, and yet he was simply putting this down to stats. I was very disappointed in him, since he'd been very supportive, and I'd believed this was because he cared. I volunteered myself to his other patients if they wanted to speak with me, and he declined on their behalf. *What a waste*, I thought.

Mid-December was the target date for my complete recovery, and just before we were due to go on holiday in the Caribbean I had an appointment with the doctor where he pronounced me clear. "You may as well forget you've ever been ill," were his precise words. Again I volunteered my phone number to his other patients, but again he declined. It occurred to me that this man had recommended surgery and a colostomy bag for me only nine months before this day. And now he was saying I may as well forget I was ever ill. And there were other patients of his going for the surgical option whom he'd denied the chance to even speak with me … or more importantly, to have a chat with Geoffrey.

This greatly saddened me and was the original reason for me to write this book, albeit that it's almost thirteen years later now! Let me say that the gastroenterologist in London was a very nice guy, but I was very disappointed in his glib statement that I was a statistical phenomenon. We had only seen *any* improvement when I started with Geoffrey's treatment. And at the same time, I'd dropped everything else, including diets, drugs, and other potions.

That holiday in Barbados was amazing. I was part of the human race again. But there was another challenge. Over the past eighteen months, I'd had all sorts of do-gooding, interfering relatives ask how I was. Now that I was well again, I was sensitive to their questions, since my answer was that I was completely fine. Now you'd have thought that people would be happy to hear that. But no! Many of them were aghast and said it was impossible and that I must be mistaken! Their doctors had said it was incurable and it would come back. Can you believe it! Some people are remarkably stupid when it comes to other people's health. Fancy saying that to anyone!

Although I was clinically better from ulcerative colitis, I was still psychologically very fragile. The fear of a relapse or of getting caught short was still very much there, and that would only be eradicated with time. I needed time to build up my confidence, time to completely trust the recovery. Remember, this had all been accomplished with words. There were no magic pills or potions. This is something that I discussed at length with Geoffrey. Remember, I'd been pretty much incontinent for over a year before I met him, and it would take at least a year of being completely well for me to have full confidence in myself again. I was nervous about going to the movie theaters for a good year after my recovery. Intestinal problems are a real prison sentence, and I understand all the mental anguish that goes alongside these conditions, as well as the obvious physical torment.

People doubting my recovery didn't help! Some even took the trouble to phone me to say that I must prepare myself to be ill again! You can imagine what I told them to do! As you can tell, I had a real attitude about this whole thing, and that's the type of attitude you can adopt too if it works for you. It worked for me, and I can only assume it will work for others. Remember, I had no frame of reference to model myself on. I knew no one who'd had what I'd had and got better from it. You're reading about my story. You now know me. You can use me as your own frame of reference.

Geoffrey had his own take on the situation, and as usual, he was right. And thankfully, I listened. He said that although I was clinically well, I had to be prepared for the odd blip before eventually the blips too would evaporate. Each blip would be less and less severe and less and less frequent until they didn't even happen anymore. Although I didn't want to hear this, it was invaluable advice for what was to occur in March of 1996.

When we came back from Barbados it was time for me to get back to work. Mission accomplished, I could now get back to a normal life.

During my sabbatical, I hadn't been completely idle. I'd completed some financial exams to complement my existing qualifications and decided to go for my dream job in the financial district of London.

In mid-January of 1996, I'd lined up an interview for a great position as a property company analyst with a major investment bank. This meant I would be analyzing the financial fortunes of REITs (Real Estate Investment Trusts) and property development companies. I went to my first interview and hit a home run. The following day I received a phone call to tell me I'd gotten the job and I just needed to be patient and wait to meet my future colleagues. Naively, I asked what I should do about my other interviews. The answer was, "Drop them. We want you. You'll be starting in the middle of March." Naively, I did just that … without ever seeing a contract.

At first I was just happy to have something lined up. This was a very reputable and large investment bank. It didn't ever occur to me that they'd do anything underhanded. Besides, I was speaking with my interviewer, who was head of the department, on a weekly basis, and he was quite reassuring. As March approached, though, I started to get concerned. Still I hadn't been asked to sign anything. My fears were allayed when my interviewer told me I'd be coming in for a meeting with my future colleagues in two weeks. In the meantime, Kelly and I organized a skiing vacation for the first week of March. Something didn't feel quite right, though. The bank's attitude had changed ever so subtly, and I could sense it. Unfortunately, so could my guts. During the skiing trip I was clinically fine, but I was certainly fragile, and I could sense something not quite right in my tummy region.

By the time I had the meeting in the bank, I was getting very wobbly. I could tell that I was on the verge of a serious relapse. The urgency and frequency had returned, and I was getting very nervous. The bank's behavior was seriously affecting my confidence in all sorts of ways, and I was feeling it in the worst possible way.

I had been told that the meeting was to be a rubber stamping of my appointment and confirming the details and structure of my employment. Imagine my surprise then when, sitting in the meeting room, I could hear these words: "I'm supposed to be meeting some chap called Guy. I don't even know what it's for." My heart sank. That meeting progressed without alarm, though it was clear that it wasn't so much a meeting as an interview. It was followed by two more that seemed to go fine. In the days that followed, my stomach area really began to get shaky. Then I got the call. The bank had decided not to employ me after all. And of the three interviewers, it was the "nicest" one who had decided to turn me down.

March–May 1996—The Blip

I instinctively knew what the implications of this would be. My confidence had taken a battering, my stomach was now doing cartwheels, and I knew I was heading for a full-scale relapse. And although I was frightened, I somehow knew (or wanted to believe) that this time it didn't have to take six months to put it right. But in the meantime, the relapse took me right back to the worst of the symptoms—incontinence, bleeding, discomfort, and agonizing pain.

I consulted with Geoffrey intensely again. And I also rethought my career plans. I never wanted to be treated in that way ever again. There was only one way to ensure that it never happened again, and that was to do an MBA. I was already well qualified, but an MBA would propel me to a new level and at a young age too. Kelly went mad! My parents weren't keen either, but my mind was set. I had four weeks to get on the course to start in October. Within days I was at an interview, preparing for a GMAT exam in June, and flinging myself into this new direction. In May I got the offer to enroll in City University's finance MBA program for 1996/97.

Almost overnight my symptoms started to improve. This time it didn't take six months to get back to normal. It took six weeks. Wow! How amazing was that. Again, I had worked closely with Geoffrey, but this time I had the inner confidence to know I could do it. After all, I'd done it before, so why not again? As Geoffrey had said, this was a blip,, and each blip thereafter would be less and less severe and less and less frequent, until eventually there would be no more blips at all.

June 1996 →→→

That was pretty much my only blip. Sure, I had the odd upset tummy after that, but nothing like that big blip. I never had any bleeding or incontinence—nothing like that again.

And so I attended the MBA course, and my career changed direction. Since that time I have enjoyed many of life's experiences. I went through a divorce, career challenges, heartbreak, bereavement— all the things that make the ups and downs of life. And never were my guts affected again. By the time I'd completely finished the MBA in 1997, I'd also completely recaptured my confidence and could take my good health for granted. It was accomplished with no drugs, no diets, and no treatments whatsoever. As Geoffrey had promised, I could take my good health for granted. That's not to say I'd abuse it, just that I didn't need to think about it anymore. So I didn't.

As I mentioned before, the psychological fragility and fear lasted for about a year beyond the actual physical recovery. But week by week, month by month, it too eased as my confidence rose and rose. People started to hear about me via friends and family, and I'd receive phone calls from complete strangers. I always tried to help. But they often seemed disappointed when they realized that it wasn't some sort of magic pill that I'd taken.

Even in my darkest days I realized that there was only one person who could get me well, and that was me. Somehow I'd put it there, and somehow I had to get rid of it. People would say, "You shouldn't blame yourself." I wasn't. I was merely taking responsibility for it. Because by taking responsibility for it, I was empowering myself to get rid of it too. By blaming everything around me for it, I would be disempowering myself. So it made sense to take charge of the situation, and then I got lucky by meeting Geoffrey. But it's my firm belief that once I'd set the target, I'd have found someone else ... eventually! The fact that it was Geoffrey is a massive bonus, but I trusted him from the outset, and he's such a great guy. Even now at eighty-three he is one of my best friends. He shares my rather immature sense of humor, and we frequently have lunch, enjoy a few drinks, and smoke his pipes! It's not what you'd call conventional therapy, but look what he enabled me to do. He gave my life back to me, and for that I will always remember him with gratitude and affection.

It's now time to share this story. It's something about which I've procrastinated for many years. Recounting my darkest days here was not something I was relishing, and that's why I chose not to recall them in the most vivid detail.

This book is about hope. It's about rousing you to believe that you too can achieve something that many people considered to be impossible. This is not about indulging in suffering. It's about setting a new mindset and inspiring you to new heights. I accomplished my miracle despite the medical profession and others effectively writing me off. I don't blame them for that. That's what they were trained to say, given the condition I had and the knowledge they had. And that's the key. Different people in different professions acquire different knowledge from different sources. Geoffrey had acquired the specific knowledge, experience, and wisdom that helped to cure me. Now, through my own personal experience, I have acquired that knowledge firsthand. With the benefit of hindsight, my miracle wasn't really a miracle. It's only called a miracle because the so-called experts said it wasn't possible. But it was possible, and I did it. Now it's your turn.

In Part 2 we're going to identify the structure of my recovery and how you can replicate that structure for yourself. I believe my recovery was measurable from my very first visit to Geoffrey. My job is to identify it so you can replicate it. Of course, I cannot personally guarantee the same results. But I do believe my results can be replicated by using the methods outlined here and modeling what I did. The vital thing here is your attitude, and you must take action. I had a real attitude about my situation, and you too need to adopt that same fighting spirit. You need to make a *decision* and *commitment* to get well and seize control of the situation. I'm going to be teaching you a *proactive* process here.

With me, the fighting spirit was always there. What Geoffrey did was to harness it in the most relaxed and effective way. See the difference between the second recovery and the first. Six weeks versus six months! Can you imagine how much more confidence that gave me into understanding the nature of the condition? It meant that no matter what challenges were materializing, I now knew with confidence how to overcome them and retain my health.

If anyone tells you it's impossible, remember my story. You have a frame of reference that I never had until I created it for myself.

Now let's go to Part 2, where we'll examine some of what I consider to be myths about IBD conditions. After that we'll go through the structure of how to create a healthier future for yourself.

Addendum

I want to share with you two instances of how a perceived relapse can occur, and how you can deal with it. We're talking about a time after you're fully better again but where your subconscious mind may bring up some issues for you.

Recurring Themes in Your Life

Many years after I was fully fit again, I had a business situation where I had created a project that was incredibly exciting to me. Because my background was finance, I needed people around me who were in this other field of expertise. To cut a long story short, I invited a friend of mine, who subsequently recommended her partner's involvement. And that's where it all went badly wrong!

Not only was this man's consultation completely counterproductive, but he also possessed a highly aggressive bullying streak in a project that was 100 percent mine! Suddenly a project that I had devised, nurtured, and copyrighted was being hijacked by someone who was threatening me at every turn while my friend simply stood by and watched.

This would be intolerable at the best of times, but for the first time in years, I felt serious discomfort and urgency in my intestines again. That was it. Nothing and no one was going to affect me in such a way. I called in the lawyers … and the business problem was solved. And before undertaking the legal solution, I also saw Geoff, just once, and the physical problem was solved.

Now, how was that achieved? Well, incredibly simply. Talking under hypnosis, I recalled that this nasty scenario bore many of the hallmarks where I'd felt intensely emotionally bullied and outnumbered in the past. My subconscious had mistakenly lumped the experiences together, and I guess in an attempt to alert me, it had triggered the same emotional and chemical responses ... in my gut. Once my subconscious had the opportunity to express itself, the physical problem disappeared ... in twenty-four hours!

This experience was a massive learning experience for many reasons. First, I realized how fast the physical problem could disappear if you can get your mind right. Second, I learned more about the precise nature of how stress can affect one's health. You see, there's a lot of stress that we can all cope with and it will not affect us. But if an event reminds our subconscious of a deeply rooted emotional scar, then a seemingly small incident can have significant physical ramifications until such time that the subconscious has a chance to express itself. Once that's done, the emotional blockage is released, and the fit body is restored again.

A very similar experience happened also when I was involved romantically with a wonderful woman but found myself in a situation that was hugely reminiscent of certain highly emotionally intense events in my relationship with Kelly. Again, the discomfort appeared quite severely, and again, once my subconscious had communicated the issue with me, I was able to confront the issue and the physical problem evaporated.

These two experiences were very short-term blips (not full relapses) on a landscape of otherwise perfectly uninterrupted good health. It is no coincidence that the subconscious was able to communicate the reasons for the issues, and once communicated, my body was able to return to normal.

If you're reading this and wondering what this means in practical terms, it's very simple. For our purposes, the hypnotic experience is optimized if you yourself are involved in the dialogue. This is for two reasons. First, it typically means your brain will be at the optimum (alpha state) frequency and not too deep. Second, it enables your subconscious to express itself in its truest sense. This is often enough to clear the underlying problem. And all we're interested in is the end prize—our complete good health.

PART TWO—The Roadmap

Myths and Dangerous Suggestions

Before we get into the mechanics of my recovery, it's important to highlight the things I was told in journals or by people who supposedly cared about me! I don't want you to be irresponsible, but I do want you to be careful about what you give credence to. Many general and glib comments out there exist without any sound empirical evidence to back up the statements in the first place. Now some skeptics may say that my story can't be called empirical per se, but I will stand up anywhere and tell my story. Besides, it's all documented in my medical notes anyway. I was always careful to tell my doctor what I was doing with alternative treatments so he could monitor my progress at all times. I never stopped getting the check-ups until the thing had disappeared for good in the spring of 1996.

Myth—"It's in the genes."

It is not in the genes! No one in my family has had it—not my direct family nor my indirect family. When I was first diagnosed, the doctors told me it was genetic. When I told them that no one in my immediate family had it, their response was, "Well, there must be someone like a distant cousin who's had it. Check out your family history."

Well, excuse me! Surely if I have to look that far away in my family tree, then it cannot really be a genetic thing. Otherwise lots of other family members would have had it too! And they don't. I felt really patronized by this attitude. It was clearly an attempt to find an easy reason to identify as the cause, and it was complete nonsense.

Myth—"It's incurable."

Clearly this is not the case, at least not with me. Remember that when a doctor makes a statement, it is his or her opinion only, not a statement of fact. Just consider that only a few hundred years ago the world was flat ... apparently! Doctors are a wonderful part of modern society. However, they are not gods, and they only know what they are taught. So far, the medical profession has been rather unsuccessful with two major areas of the body, namely the intestine and the skin (epidermis). To me, it's a natural trait to never give in ... ever! So when doctors told me there was no cure, I took it to mean "from the doctors' perspective." Therefore I simply had to look elsewhere!

How many times have you heard that someone only had weeks to live, and yet there they are, still alive years later? How many times have you heard of a woman being told she can't conceive, and then months later she's pregnant? These things happen on a daily basis. Again, I have the utmost respect for doctors, but they too can be wrong, and they're not gods.

I remember one time I was up in Scotland meeting an old work friend a few years after I got well. He was engaged to a medic. Over dinner he told her my story, and she then gave me her own interrogation. She was not just stunned about it but was actually angry! My recovery went against everything she had been taught about colitis, and she literally put her hands around my neck at the dinner table, shaking me and saying it couldn't be true! I have to say part of me did find it funny, but the other part was angry. Why couldn't she be happy about what was an amazing story? Why was being right so much more important to her than someone's health? Sadly, this is the way a lot of people think. Years later I look back on that dinner with great amusement, and it's given me a great anecdote to tell. But I do want to add that a number of other doctor friends of mine were and have always been wholly supportive and accepting of what I did, without questioning it.

As you start to make tangible improvements, you'll have to be slightly careful of people who are skeptics or who seem to delight in other people's illness. Just ignore them. They're simply not worth the bother. That's a lesson that took me a good couple of years to heed.

Myth—"It never goes away."

Again, I don't really need to elaborate on this one. It can, it does, and given the right approach, it will go away completely. I know I'm not the only one who's gotten rid of it. I wasn't the first, and I won't be the last.

As an additional point, I hate the word remission. In my book, it's either there or it isn't. In my case, it hasn't been there for nine years. The word remission has a nasty connotation about it, and that's why I will never use the word. Remember, it was words that got me better, so I'm selective now about the words I choose to communicate with myself and others. Words are very powerful, as you're probably discovering in this course.

Dangerous Suggestion—
"It can lead to other diseases."

For me, this is one of the most harmful suggestions, and in my opinion, it is simply not backed up by enough statistical evidence. Remember, I was told it was genetic and that I couldn't get better, and look what happened there. Remember I was told it would never go away, and look what happened there too.

The reality is that people *can* live to a ripe old age with IBD, colitis, or Crohn's, and they do. In my case, I didn't want to be suffering all that time, so I went and sought ways of getting rid of it. I really don't think the medical profession truly understands the nature of IBD conditions, and that's why they're generally poor at treating them. So far the medical profession has come up with a few drugs that can mask some of the symptoms in some cases, some of the time, and a whole load of generalizations as to why it can't be cured. What they mean is, "Why we haven't found our own cure yet." People have gotten better from this. You just have to take them, and me, as the examples you follow.

The power of suggestion is what got me well again. So people really need to take more care about the words they use and the words the pay attention to.

The Winning Attitude

As I mentioned before, I had a real attitude about getting better. Throughout the illness, I was inundated with unwanted opinions from people who were more interested in peddling their viewpoint and being right than actually being helpful or constructive. The vast majority simply didn't think I had a prayer of getting better, so they tried to manage my expectations, suggesting that I learn to live with the problem. I would promptly tell them that *they* could live with it if they wanted, but I wasn't going to!

Help Groups

I was advised to join various help and support groups, including the Crohn's and Colitis Foundation of America and the United Kingdom equivalent. I politely declined. The person concerned asked why not. I replied, "I don't want to be around a bunch of ill people!" (I know that was harsh of me, but do hear me out on this one!)

"Well, you're one of them," he exclaimed. "You're in the same boat as them."

"But I don't want to be in the same boat as them. I don't want to be one of them," I replied. "I want to be in the boat with people who have recovered from it."

"There are no such people. There isn't such a boat."

"Fine, I'll just have to make my own boat then!" (Please note that there were plenty of expletives in my diction that I've deleted here!)

The point was simple. I did not accept that I couldn't get better, and that was my attitude from the very beginning. The more people who told me I couldn't do it, the more resolved I was to prove them wrong.

As you can imagine, I didn't make too many friends throughout this experience. All I wanted was to get better. Nothing else mattered to me. And because I had no one else to copy, I simply had to make it up as I was going along.

About a year after I'd gotten better, around 1997, my attitudes had softened considerably. In my desire to do some good, I did actually contact the Crohn's and Colitis Foundation of America (CCFA) to tell them my story. Disappointingly, they were only interested in what drugs had helped me. When I explained the nature of treatment I'd received, they simply weren't interested at all. I asked them why not, to which they said they were only interested in drug therapies. This simply confirmed my original decision not to attend any of their programs.

My attitude was further hardened when a cousin of mine asked if I'd like to attend a CCFA charity dinner in New York. Of course I was interested. It was suggested that I could even say a few words. When I said that I could tell the attendees about my story and how I'd gotten better, he explained point blank that it would not be well received, so I declined the invitation. I was stupefied. How could my story not be well received at a function crammed with people (and their partners) who were still suffering from something that I had gotten rid of?

When you combine these anecdotes with the fact that the specialist in London didn't want to even have a chat with Geoffrey, having witnessed my recovery firsthand, how can anyone be surprised at my attitude toward the establishment? Surely an organization like CCFA should be interested in anyone or any method or any story that contains success within it? No, not even them.

So, as you can now see, my journey was a lonely one, and my attitude about it put many backs up! Looking back nine years later, I can afford a wry smile about it all. And there were some friends at the time who were incredibly supportive. If you remember that they had no frames of reference for a cure for colitis, it's all the more phenomenal that certain friends chose to back my efforts to the hilt.

Small Words, Special Effects

I remember back in April/May 1995, pretty much at my worst and with me being stick thin, I had to speak with one of my superior bosses, who I didn't really know very well, as he worked in a different building. I told him that if I wasn't substantially better within a month, then I would leave the firm. I didn't want them carrying me as they had up to then. I was in a highly sociable job, and I couldn't even go out for drinks because of my condition and the restrictions I had been put under.

The boss said this: "Well, Guy, if anyone can get better from this, it's you." That was it. I can't tell you how special those words were. I didn't even know or care if he meant them! They were very powerful and special words. OK, I didn't make any improvements for that next month and so left the firm ... and fatefully phoned Geoffrey only days after leaving. But the point is, as much as people can kill with words, some people have a knack of choosing the right words and delivering them in a very powerful and memorable way.

I did mention some of my friends and how phenomenal they were. A more junior boss in the firm and his wife became my best friends during this period. At a time where I was basically incontinent, I wasn't much fun to be around or have around! Accordingly, I did struggle to get out for a while. Yet this couple, Dominic and Lulu, would insist that Kelly and I go round to their place for dinner at least once a week. I would say, "But I'll just be on the loo the whole night," to which they replied, "Well, at least it's a different loo. You're still coming over!" How can you describe that sort of compassion? They're my best friends to this very day.

So I did have some wonderful support, even if it did turn out to be from more unlikely sources. They never once questioned my commitment or ability to do something extraordinary; it was never even a consideration. They accepted what I was doing and encouraged me. It only takes a couple of people to say the right things to melt away all the negative nonsense being peddled by others. I paid utmost attention to the good guys and used my natural instincts as a polarity responder to vow to prove all the others wrong! What that says about my personality, who knows! But that kind of bulldog spirit sure came in handy in that dilemma.

"Disappointment Requires Adequate Planning"

Richard Bandler has a saying: "Disappointment requires adequate planning." If you think about it, it makes perfect sense. Many people literally prepare themselves for disappointment, for arguments that aren't ever going to happen, and for let-downs that never materialize. If someone sneezes in the same room as them, they'll immediately start fantasizing about the cold they think they'll get! You must adopt the opposite approach. Prepare your mind for a wonderful life, being totally fit. Remember what I did. I celebrated my recovery even when I was at my worst, well before I even met Geoffrey. I prepared myself and my mind for the recovery I would make. And so must you.

Secondary Gains

You must participate and be fully involved in your own recovery and want it more than anything else. You must be honest with yourself about what you're doing and how you're thinking.

Many people, when they get a medical condition, use it as a crutch and get comfortable within that condition very easily. Having a medical condition such as those we're talking about here can give people the excuse not to go places or to behave in a certain way that would otherwise be unacceptable. On the other hand, some people find that their medical complaints make them the center of attention, and that's all they ever talk about! This is called a secondary gain. In other words it's a perceived gain, but in actual fact it is predicated by a losing situation in the first place (i.e., being ill). Why have to be ill in order to get out of going to a party? Why not just say no? Why not just be honest? Being honest will eliminate any perceived need for any secondary gains.

My symptoms led me to be slightly agoraphobic. I was frightened of leaving the house because I was basically incontinent. It became very distressing for me to contemplate being more than one minute away from a toilet for any length of time. Therefore, I associated going out with that distress, and so the spiral continued. This is why, even when I was better, it took a while for the mental fragility to evaporate. I remember going to the movies was particularly difficult, but that too went away once I got my confidence back.

Secondary gains are a common psychological phenomenon but would not exist if people were completely honest with themselves. Be aware of this phenomenon, and be honest with yourself. I've met so many people over the last nine years who contacted me to hear how I became well again. When I told them, they were disappointed that I wasn't simply naming a magic bullet that would cure them overnight. And yet what I was describing to them had so much more potential and proof of success than anything else they were contemplating.

This is the type of conversation I've had with countless people over the years.

"Hello, Guy, I've heard about you from a friend, and I really want to know how you got better, etc."

So I'd ask them a few questions and tell them very succinctly that I'd tried a number of approaches but the only one that had any real impact, and actually got me completely better too, was Geoffrey's treatment.

"Oooooh, I don't want to do hypnosis. I won't do that!"

"Why not?" I'd ask.

"I don't want someone controlling my brain."

I've heard this time and time again. As I mentioned before, there are two ways to handle this statement. The reality is that Geoffrey's style of treatment and hypnotherapy teaches you how to think and control your own brain. He doesn't control it. He teaches you to do it for yourself. The other way of dealing with such comments is to say that it might not be a bad idea for someone else to control their brain in order for them to get well anyway!

It basically boils down to two things: honesty and how much you want it. I was always intrigued by hypnosis anyway. Nothing about it scared me. Everything about it fascinated me. And if it exposed my deepest, darkest secrets, who cares! I just wanted to get better. Nothing else mattered. I didn't care if that meant I had to change. If it meant I had my health back, you bet I'd change for that!

Many people simply don't want it as much as I did. They're prepared to compromise. I wasn't prepared to do that. From the time I walked out of that hospital in Portland, I was a man on a mission. Nothing other than a complete recovery was going to be good enough for me. And that became my obsession from then on. Fortunately, now that I've done it and have been well for so long, you don't have to adopt the manic approach that I did. All you have to do is ask yourself how much you want it and what you're prepared to do about it.

Some basic research will show you that hypnotherapy is perfectly safe. All you need to do is find the right person—someone you can trust, someone whose ability you have faith in, someone who *knows* they can help you. Those are the ingredients I looked for. The woman in that first session I had was probably perfectly competent, but I didn't have the belief in her. So I called Geoffrey instead, and the rest is history.

Please do what you can to make yourself comfortable with this approach. My story alone should accomplish that for you. I firmly believe that those people who shy away from what has proved to be a winning formula simply don't want it enough to be fit and well again. If you really want it, you'll try anything. And making a few adjustments to your thought process while someone's talking to you—that's not much to ask for, is it?

Let me also say this. You will still be the same person. Your basic characteristics won't change. What may change is your interpretation and reaction to various things. My hunger to succeed and do well wasn't affect in the slightest. If anything, I became hungrier because I had proved that I was capable of extraordinary things. And so are you too. Things that used to bother me and get me all upset started to become little nuisances instead. That didn't mean I was an automaton with no feelings. Far from it. I was still just as sentimental as ever, if not more so because of the emotion of the entire experience. But I was able to put things in context and cope far better. I had learned how to think in a more constructive manner. I now had much better thinking habits. I wasn't arguing with myself in my mind any more. I wasn't planning adequately for disappointment any more! And that led to sustained improvements until I was back to normal again.

Common Denominators

There are several common denominators that many people with gut problems seem to share. In my experience, these are behavioral traits more than anything else. And I can relate to those personality traits too.

This is a difficult section, and I've gotten in trouble when speaking with people in the past because within minutes I can often nail exactly how people think, what they say to themselves, what they're thinking about, and even whom they're thinking about! This all gets very personal, but keep in mind that the only thing that matters is that you get well again.

Thinking Habits

Go into your mind and listen. Really listen carefully. How do you think in general? Are thoughts all jumbled in your mind, racing around at the speed of light? Is there a lot of noise in your mind? Do you have too many things going on all at once? Do you have the same kind of looping thoughts going round and round in your mind, almost as if they're beyond your control?

Looping Destructive Thoughts

We'll cover this in more detail later in this section, but one of the key common denominators is this issue of looping negative (or destructive) thoughts. This is when the same kind of damaging thought pattern keeps looping over and over again, seemingly beyond your conscious perception and seemingly out of your control.

Typically these thoughts stem from anger and originate from a highly judgmental perspective.

These thoughts often entail preparatory rehearsals for future conflicts and negative encounters that haven't happened and which may never actually happen. But your mind runs off at a tangent, preparing you for a whole host of negative outcomes that could possibly happen. It's like a survival mechanism, but it's actually very destructive.

Anger

The looping negative thoughts often have anger at their root. The vast majority of people I've met with Crohn's, colitis, and IBS were able to recognize this anger, which is the first step in diffusing it. The anger and the looping thoughts feed off each other. The more you indulge in the negative looping thoughts, the angrier you become. The angrier you become, the more you indulge in the destructive looping thoughts. Diffuse the anger and the self-arguments become redundant and unnecessary. Eliminate the looping thoughts and there's less to be angry about. It's a bit of a chicken and egg situation. What we need to do is reverse the damaging habits and replace them with a virtuous cycle of healthy thinking.

Being Overly Judgmental

Some people will argue that everyone is judgmental or making judgments all the time. That's true to an extent, but as with so many things in life, moderation is the key.

Of course, most people have opinions, and that's healthy. It's also healthy to have passion in life. The problem occurs when you have strong opinions about everything, even things that barely matter to you. This can turn into excessive judgmental thinking, which (a) uses up a lot of energy and (b) is a typical component of a destructive looping thought pattern.

Observe subjectively if you're over-opinionated and angry about something in particular. It may not be easy to admit, but you must be honest with yourself if you want to make progress and get on the road to recovery.

A Thought Travels

It's commonly accepted now that thoughts have a frequency. You can actually measure a thought. As such, thoughts actually *travel*. They have a beginning, they make their journey, and then they either loop around or fade into another thought that then begins the process all over. The problem is that destructive, negative looping thoughts can go round and round and round in an almost never-ending fashion. If they are allowed to continue in the conscious mind, a strong habit is formed, and the destructive looping thought is then embedded into the subconscious, almost like an undetected computer Trojan virus.

The problem is that, not only does this destructive cycle of thought lead to wild emotional swings, but then it also leads to nasty physical consequences, often appearing in the gut.

We've all had experiences whereby a thought made us *feel* something different in our bodies. One of the most common thought-body experiences is having butterflies in our stomachs because of nerves. Well, multiply the intensity of the nerves a few thousand times, keep it going for months on end, and instead of butterflies in you stomach, you're dealing with a herd of angry elephants! And that's what gives rise to these types of severe intestinal issues such as Crohn's, colitis, and to a less severe extent, IBS.

The origins of the physical problem are in the thinking routines, and that can be very subtle indeed. The horrendous physical effects of this destructive looping thought routine are there for all to see.

Thoughts Spark Chemical and Hormonal Reactions

There's a further issue in all of this. The negative thinking patterns create a chemical or hormonal reaction, which in itself seems to be quite addictive. And the easiest way to produce this "drug" is for the destructive thoughts to keep looping away.

The brain is made up of billions of nerve cells known as neurons. Neurons connect together via tentacles called dendrites (the signal receivers) and axon terminals (the transmitters) at lightning speed, hence our ability to react so fast to internal and external stimuli.

When neurons connect in this way, they don't actually touch per se. There is a gap, and this gap is called a synapse. This is where the electrical charge occurs as impulses are transmitted from one neuron to the next via the synapses of the dendrites and axon terminals.

Some studies suggest that a single neuron can have as many as 1,000 to 10,000 synapses (or more!), meaning it can communicate with thousands of other neurons at the same time. Now when you consider the brain has literally billions of neurons, the permutations and combinations become literally mind-boggling. It also means our brains have almost infinite capacity for storing information, learning concepts, and creating instructions to the body.

Each firing of these electrical impulse signals creates a unique awareness in perception to each individual, either consciously or sub-consciously. In other words, we are able to create associations with each experience. Such is our brain's capacity that we can create unlimited associations. For example, if you smell the perfume of your first partner, you'll literally feel that pang of nostalgia as you smell the fragrance even many years later. Each association we create has its own unique neural pathway, bringing an array of chemical and hormonal reactions that enable us to *feel* or have an emotional reaction ranging from imperceptible to out-of-control.

A strong belief comes about by the maintenance of a specific neural pathway. Think of a chalk line on a tennis court—that would be akin to an idea. An idea can be easily painted over or worn away. Now imagine the chalk line is dug into the tennis court about twelve inches deep all the way around the court, and now you have something more like a belief—more difficult to make a mini-trench disappear than a line, but still possible.

Now think of a destructive looping thought pattern that runs and runs over and over again. It's more like that twelve-inch deep mini-trench, but again, do be assured, it's possible to fill it in and replace it with something far more constructive.

Our thoughts are generated by whatever set of neurons are firing at any one time. It's possible for one person to associate dogs as friendly pets and another person to associate them as dangerous animals. A belief can be formed by a single experience. The stronger the emotional reaction at the time, or the more it is repeated, the deeper the imprint on the conscious and subconscious will be.

A looping destructive thinking pattern may have been encouraged by a single event or repetitive events that caused the need to create a survival mechanism. The problem is compounded when that destructive thinking pattern ingrains itself and digs its own trench in the mind, literally embedding itself as a constant and active neural pathway.

This in turn produces the chemical and hormonal reactions that eventually lead to the gut reacting in severe fashion. As mentioned earlier, the irony is that the chemical reactions caused by the destructive looping thoughts are seemingly addictive in themselves. With the body inadvertently craving the drug, it's as if the mind is fooled into repeating the destructive thinking habit, and thus the vicious cycle keeps looping.

So, what's the answer? Well, eliminate the destructive looping thought habit, and you'll also get rid of the destructive chemical reaction. With that gone the gut will have a chance to heal.

With the brain being akin to an electrical circuit, the negative thought patterns use up terrific amounts of energy resources, and it's not uncommon for destructive-pattern thinkers to have issues with their energy levels. When the repetitive negative thoughts are banished, it follows that higher energy levels are restored.

So, how do we get rid of the looping thought habit? We get rid of them by using techniques that lead to *you* taking control of your thoughts. These techniques include behavioral techniques (consciously interrupting negative thought cycles with the rhetorical questions), hypnotic guided meditations, and learning how to breathe deeply with more control.

The very act of breathing with control will help you control your thoughts, actions, and change your body chemistry for the better. Controlled breathing is one of the core principles of meditation and yoga, which are universally accepted as being beneficial to our mental and physical health. Add a simple mantra such as "I am in control" to each slow out-breath and you're then establishing control over your breathing and thinking at the same time. Do that for ten long, deep, slow breaths, and then increase to twenty. Sounds easy ... try it!

Your Breathing

How do you breathe? Is it too shallow? Try to develop an awareness of these things. Once you're conscious of these things, if you sense that they're not necessarily the healthiest way of thinking, you can start to effect conscious change, which in turn can supplement the unconscious alterations that can also be benefiting you in the background. We're devising a multi-pronged assault on the issues here so we can be as effective and efficient in getting back to full fitness.

We all communicate with ourselves through our internal dialogue. How do you communicate with yourself? What do you hear yourself saying to yourself? How do you say these things with yourself? Are you nice to yourself, or do you berate yourself and others constantly in your mind? I'll permit one exception, and that's the occasional surrender to road rage! But I only mean occasional, like say twice a year!

Just like breathing more deeply and steadily, these seemingly small and unrelated issues can have profound effects on your health when you make the necessary adjustments. Take them seriously, be aware of them, and if you catch yourself communicating with yourself in a destructive way, simply ask yourself if that's a particularly smart thing for you to be doing. Ask yourself if it's doing you any good. And then you might start to smile just a bit and playfully shrug your shoulders, realizing that you simply don't need to go around self-flagellating all the time!

You're now starting the process of healthier thinking. And with it, you can add some healthy breathing too. We'll talk more about that a little later, but be aware of it now.

Family and Relationships

Warning! This can be a sensitive area. You'd be surprised how many people with bowel disorders have such similarities, it's astonishing. Many have serious issues going on (at least in their minds) with their families or closest personal relationships. By families we're talking parents, siblings, or very close relatives. By personal relationships we're talking husbands, wives, girlfriends, boyfriends, and even work colleagues in some cases.

Everyone has some form of self-communication. This means we all effectively talk to ourselves! This doesn't mean we're mad … yet! It's not that we all talk to ourselves; it's the *way* in which we do so that will influence our mental state and sometimes our physical state. It's a very real phenomenon that many people with bowel disorders have some serious issues, at least in their mind, with their family and relationships.

They somehow get into the habit of role-playing in their minds, typically playing out scenes of confrontation regarding events that often haven't even happened. This is gross insecurity, possibly fostered by inconsistency within the relationship. If you think about it, one of the greatest challenges a parent can have is to be consistent. When there is a real lack of consistency and you then add some volatility and high expectations into the mix, then you're potentially creating a problem in the future for the children as they grow into adulthood. This type of insecurity is borne out of relationships where:

(a) The child never feels good enough.

(b) One day the child's actions are treated one way, and the next day the same actions are treated a completely different way.

This type of inconsistency, while often unintentional from the parents, can lead to massive insecurity and lack of confidence because the child feels the subconscious need to prepare for all eventualities in his or her mind. It's a survival mechanism, if you like. If the parents are volatile in nature, then the mind preparation becomes all the more essential for the child's subconscious need to survive. The preparation will involve rehearsing all eventualities—in other words, the child will go through the arguments or confrontations in his or her mind in order to be fully prepared just in case the event happens.

This then becomes habitual, and as the child grows into an adult, the habit is deep rooted in the subconscious as the only way of handling the inconsistencies of the upbringing. Breaking a habit like this requires some skill and work with the subconscious mind. It's easy enough and is made even easier when you're aware of it consciously, because then you can catch yourself doing it and put a stop to it as it starts. The more you stop yourself doing it, the nearer you are to putting a stop to it even beginning in the first place. Then you add the rhetorical questioning technique (What good is this behavior doing me? etc.) and you'll break the negative cycle.

Inconsistency as a parent is not a crime. It's not evil—but it can be very damaging, particularly for sensitive children, because it can lead to this kind of self-destructive thinking pattern into their teens and young adulthood. It is no coincidence that the common age for bowel disorders is from late teens to mid twenties. This is where we're going through a lot of changes in terms of developing our minds, and longstanding bad thinking habits have quietly gained way too much power by that phase of our lives because they're constantly running in the background, almost like a computer virus.

This is the part that many people find very difficult to accept. No one really likes to admit that they may have the issues I've just outlined. I can pretty much tell from someone's voice what is going on with them. Sometimes I'll take a chance and tell them straight away, and their reaction is always extreme. Remember, I'm not a professional therapist; I'm just someone who went through an extreme case but got over it completely. I understand. I paid attention to what was going on and was completely honest with myself. So must you be. If you truly want to be better, then it's simply a process you have to go through.

If we're talking about the inconsistency of relatives like we've just discussed, there's no point in recriminating. As I said, it's not necessarily intentional. Consistency is one of human beings' greatest challenges. Unfortunately, inconsistency of behavior can leave others in a mess.

Please take the time to consider if you fit into this category. Really look into your mind to contemplate how you think and how you communicate with yourself every day. Think about your personal relationships. You may not be able to change them, but you can certainly change the way you react to them.

People would ask me years later whether my marriage, which eventually failed, had anything to do with my getting ill in the first place. My answer is considered. Perhaps, in becoming committed into a doomed relationship, I exposed myself to a catalyst. Perhaps. However, that would be doing a massive disservice to Kelly, and besides, I was still fully committed to the relationship when I got well, so that theory really doesn't quite follow. I understand the issues to be much deeper than that. I had lived with my bad thinking habits since I was a child, and they had become progressively worse and worse over the years. Bad thinking can eventually lead to bad health. That's what happened in my case. The bad thinking spiraled out of control, and I wouldn't have known about it if I hadn't become physically ill and then discovered the root of what was going on.

When I say that bad thinking *can* lead to bad health, don't let's assume it has to happen that way. There are plenty of people out there with bad thinking habits who don't have a physical health problem. Maybe it only affects the hyper-sensitive in this way. It doesn't really matter. If you're someone who can relate to this section, in a way you should be rejoicing. We can now start to unravel the insecurities and replace the bad thinking with some good thinking. The results will be profound on many levels.

Breathing

Bad thinking habits can manifest themselves in many ways. One of the most common ways is the impact they have on your stress levels, which in turn affects your breathing. We're talking cause and effect all the way here. And before you may succumb to the temptation to dismiss this, remember I was told about the breathing as a major factor by the reflexologist many months before I met with Geoff. In turn, the hypnotic phenomenon also contains breathing as one of its central components. There's no question that my breathing changed beyond all measure for the better as part of my recovery. We only really focused on it during the hypnotic inductions, but I was acutely aware of how much more relaxed I felt when I breathed more deeply and steadily.

It's a fact that most people breathe way too shallow. One of the reasons smokers gain some form of relaxation from that awful habit is because they're breathing in deeply as they inhale. Their entire physiology is changed by this. Try inhaling like a smoker but without the cigarette and see how you feel. Go on—fill up your lungs with *oxygen*—and see how it feels. I'll bet it feels different, doesn't it?

So, how can you learn to breathe more effectively? Well, for a start, be aware of it. Breathe more through your abdomen than your chest. Put one of your hands over your stomach and the other over your solar plexus. Feel the warmth of your hands and now breathe in as slowly as you possibly can. Almost let the air seep in; there's no need to suck it in. Just let it drift in very slowly and relax your shoulders as you do so. Allow your eyes to defocus, and as you reach the top of your breath, just hold it for a few seconds and then let the air out as slowly as you possibly can. If this makes you feel a bit giddy, then this is the effect of more oxygen getting into your body!

Now, obviously you can't go around breathing like that all the time. However, you should be able to get in the rhythm of breathing in a more measured way in the normal course of your day. Note how much better it feels to breathe in this way, and keep on reminding yourself about it. You're now going to be creating a new habit that will help you and contribute to your progress.

Common Denominators Summary

These are the kinds of common denominators, not necessarily exclusive, that can plague sufferers of bowel disorders. Most people I talk to are pretty forward in confirming these as their main issues. Some, however, can become defensive. No matter what the case, take a look inside and consider if any of the issues we've discussed so far (or similar issues) could be affecting your health in any way. The more honest you are with yourself, the more progress you'll make.

Also, consider your attitude and how much you really want to get better. Are you willing to compromise? I wasn't. I wanted to be completely free of any physical troubles. That was my attitude and I was prepared to keep going until I won. Remember, the key is fighting spirit aligned with the relaxed mindset.

Diets

This is not a story about diets, but it's natural to make reference to diets in the context of the subject matter.

Of course, good nutrition is a key component of your overall health. However, in term of the colitis, my real progress coincided with the start of Geoffrey's treatment. Certainly I wouldn't abuse your diet and it's always good to apply basic common sense.

I have heard firsthand of cases where people with food intolerances and allergies were able to exclude certain foodstuffs and transform their conditions, so I can't rule out this type of approach. However, it's not what did it for me, and for the purposes of this course, I have to concentrate on what I do know, and help you model what I did.

By all means, get yourself tested for allergies and food intolerances. I did. But if the other things we've mentioned so far resonate with you, then it's likely that they'll be a more likely cause and not sensitivity with food.

PART THREE—
The Step-by-Step Approach

A Replicable Methodology

The entire concept of Neuro Linguistic Programming (NLP) is based upon the premise that human behavior and outstanding achievement is replicable. We're really only interested in constructive and positive human behavior, so in this sense we're focusing on modeling excellence.

What happened with me could be described as something worth replicating for other sufferers in its own right, and it's my firm belief that what I did can be replicated by anyone. Geoffrey has had plenty of success with others who suffered like me. I wasn't the first, and I'm not the last, so this opens up the possibilities for others—like you, for example.

Let's identify and summarize the various factors that contributed to my recovery and long-term well being. Let's also examine the techniques I've learned since that time, and which I've used to transform peoples' lives in literally days.

We'll then be in a position to construct our own formula—and the results will astound you.

Attitude

o *Taking Responsibility.* My attitude to my problems was that somehow I must be responsible for putting them there, and therefore I was empowered to remove them. This is not the same as blame. I did not blame myself. I simply gave myself the power to put things right.

o *Fighting Spirit.* As much as anything that is contained in this course, I've tried to imbue you with that same fighting spirit that I had all along. You are entitled to be healthy in your life. Just because doctors say it's not possible doesn't mean it's not. It's just their opinion. If I'm a statistical phenomenon, then so can you be. We can all be statistical phenomena until we become the norm, rather than the exception.

o *Honesty.* I was completely honest with myself and was open to change. I wanted to get better, and anything that could facilitate that was acceptable to me. You must now be honest with yourself and ask how much you really want to better again. Are you willing to compromise? I wasn't. I had to be completely well again, and nothing short of that was going to be good enough for me.

o *Open Minded.* I would have tried anything to get well … and let's face it, I've already shared with you a few of the more wacky things I did try in the name of getting better! Just because you're doing hypnosis it doesn't mean you have a mental problem. Don't get all hooked up on that. It's purely a technique that enables you to learn more quickly, learn how to think more constructively for yourself, and therefore improve your general level of health all over.

I've always had a fascination with the mind. It really is all powerful. Now you can use yours for your own benefit.

o   *Relaxed, Confident, and Controlled.* You'll see and hear from the induction below how important these forces are. If you are relaxed then your body and mind will be more efficient, thereby allowing more positive energy states. You should start to nurture confidence in yourself and confidence in your ability to perform extraordinary deeds. You can feel confident in your ability to be well again. Look to the future at the pictures of yourself and see an animated, vibrant, healthy, colorful, and happy person. You can exaggerate the images, making them bigger, brighter, and clearer until you literally step into the image of yourself and join in the fun. In this way you can also be in control of yourself, your emotions, and your communications. If you are controlled in this way, then you'll feel more relaxed anyway, because you'll stop having those arguments in your own mind, you'll develop more and more confidence, and you'll be relaxed as you start to feel much better.

o   *Patience.* Once the process begins, remember about the charts and that there are no straight lines on a graph without some sort of retracement. This is the natural order of life as prescribed by the Fibonacci sequence of numbers. Life is all about progress, but progress never occurs unabated. There are always pauses and retracements. That's nature. You're using nature to make your recovery, and having made the initial leaps, the odd pause here and there is only a confirmation that you're on the right track. Keep at it and you'll make another stride forward soon.

o *Release Anger.* As mentioned earlier, if you've recognized yourself to have anger, then you need to have a quiet word with yourself and allow it to evaporate. It typically doesn't matter what the anger is about. What matters is that you get rid of it. You do this by way of the conscious thinking techniques outlined below. Ask yourself why you're feeling anger and what good it's doing you. Ask yourself if there's something more constructive you could do or feel that would help with your physical and mental state.

o *Abandon Judgment.* If you've recognized that you might be overly judgmental, then you need to stop it. Ask yourself what it would feel like to not judge constantly. Consciously free yourself from the burden of being judgmental. The pay-off will be immediate in that you'll feel clearer-minded and you'll then find that you have more energy. Being judgmental uses a lot of fuel and promotes a lot of negative energy. Abandon judgment and liberate yourself.

Applications and Techniques

There are three main techniques that should be combined that will transform habitually bad thinking. To facilitate my recovery, I used hypnosis and conscious mind techniques in order to break the destructive pattern and instill a new, permanent positive thinking pattern. These techniques were allied to the determination that was a hallmark of my commitment to being well again. Once I'd set my stall out for a full recovery, it became a question of when, not if. It was a question of discovering what was going to work. Of course, along the journey, most things I tried didn't work at all. But I gave each one a proper try before discarding it and moving onto something else until I sensed I was succeeding. My strategy involved gauging if a treatment was working. If it was I would stick with it until the job was done.

(i)   Hypnosis/Hypnotherapy

Of course, this means with a trusted, competent, and experienced therapist. Experienced does not necessarily mean old; it means competent. More importantly, you must have complete faith in whomever you choose to help you, and you must trust him or her implicitly. You should notice some adjustments in your thinking patterns within a couple of sessions, and from there, you'll start to notice that the physical manifestations of the condition are easing—or at the very least, not getting any worse!

(ii)   Conscious Thinking Techniques

In other words, the things I did to continue the good work in my own time, each day like ensuring my breathing was okay and stopping myself from getting into those destructive self-arguments by asking myself rhetorical questions. Basically, I was participating in the recovery process by consciously conditioning myself to adopt good thinking habits.

In that vein, I continued the good work with some self hypnosis too. There are plenty of books on this subject, but as a shortcut, just get your breathing right, nice and deep and steady, and allow your eyes to softly unfocus and go through the different parts of your body, imagining how they can relax as you continue breathing in that way. I often find myself partially crossing my eyes as they unfocus, and combined with deeper breathing, I find myself getting into a relaxed state easily.

(iii)   The Rewind Technique

This is something I learned several years after my recovery. This is one of the most amazing discoveries and is the key to lightning results. Put it this way—had I known about this technique, my own recovery would have taken days, not months. It's that powerful.

Just so I have your attention, here's an e-mail I received from a lady whom I treated over the phone for one hour.

Dear Guy

Just to let you know that since our session last week I've experienced some amazing results. A calmer gut (now down to two trips to the toilet instead of 10/12), a really positive state of mind and also the most delicious velvety sleep which since the birth of Sam I had despaired of ever getting back!
One of the most important things I have discovered is that I need to put just as much commitment in too! I listen to your MP3 recording every night and when I hear 'the voices' I laugh them out of existence.

I was in a 'dark space' - believe me - and now I'm definitely out into the sunshine again - it feels good!

Thanks Guy!

Tricia B :))

This lady had been chronically ill with Crohn's for over twenty years. This e-mail was the result of just one session with me over the phone a few days before.

A similar story occurred with an acute and chronically ill colitis sufferer. The combination of techniques, including the Rewind technique, led to dramatic improvements even after just one session. The Rewind technique is what enabled such a dramatic response and is now a central part of the treatment.

Hi Guy

Just a very short up-date on Tyler.

Towards the end of June 2008, Tyler reached a very bad patch with his UC. The UC consultant said that the only way forward will be a total removal of the colon and a bag. We were very fortunate to make contact with you shortly after that. The operation was planned for mid September. We were eager to start Tyler on your course, because after 14 years of no progress we were willing to try anything.

...

The good news is that they are not going to remove the colon anymore because of the progress he has made in recovering from UC.

...

We are very grateful and cannot thank you enough.

Kind Regards

Johann

The Rewind Technique was originally developed by Richard Bandler as the "Fast Phobia Cure." This is one of the most powerful discoveries made in the field of Neuro Linguistic Programming (NLP). My application of it is, up to now, unique. Crucially, the technique can be used to eliminate a chronic bad thinking pattern.

The process typically involves two people—someone qualified to instruct (say, me) and a subject (let's say you). You can also do it on yourself. Simply apply each stage, step by step. This is hugely important, so take your time.

The Rewind Technique Step by Step

If you're doing this on your own, the best way of approaching this process is to read each step and familiarize yourself with it all first. Then do the whole process at one time. You may want to read each step a few times. I'll summarize it all for you at the end anyway. Please take your time with this. This is the most important part of the book.

Step 1—Anchoring Positive States (five minutes)

In this step, we're going to remind you of times you've felt amazing positive emotions, get you to re-live them, and set a physical stimulus (pinching your thumbnail against your middle finger as if you're going to click them) right at the point of a heightened positive state.

o OK, now I want you to take a deep breath, smile and relax. This is going to be fun, and it's going to be an amazing experience for you.

  Remember a time when you felt incredibly confident, You didn't have to be saving the world or anything, just something where you were about to do something and you knew you were going to do it with absolute certainty. Go on ... remember how you felt. Remember what you saw at the time, and make the images bigger and brighter ... that's right ... and more vivid, sharper ... go on ... crank it up! Remember what you heard at the time. Make it like surround sound, in front of you, behind you, above you, below you, to the right, to the left; make it *real!* And recall the other details—how you felt, how you positioned yourself, your posture, your facial expression, and anything

66

else. Be aware of every sensation you were feeling with so much confidence. It's OK, you can smile. This is supposed to feel good!

Go on, really intensify the sights, sounds, and feelings. Multiply everything by one hundred, and just when you can't crank it up any more, pinch your thumbnail against your middle finger pad and take a deep breath. Smile … that's it … and let go, breathe out, and relax!

o OK, now you're going to remember a time where you felt overwhelming curiosity. Think about something you were completely fascinated by. You had a real passion for discovering more about this thing you were riveted by.

Go on … remember what you saw at the time, and make the images bigger and brighter … that's right … and more vivid—in front of you, to your left and right, in your peripheral vision, above and below. Even be aware of what was behind you. Make sharper images. Go on, really crank it up this time! Remember what you heard at the time. Make it like you're in a movie theater. The sounds are all around you. It's so real, you can feel like you're re-living this wonderful experience all over again … right now! And remember the other details—how you felt, your balance, your facial expressions, and anything else Be aware of every sensation you were feeling with so much curiosity. Remember, this is fun, so have fun with it. This is supposed to feel good!

Go on, really intensify the sights, sounds, and feelings. Multiply everything by a hundred, and just when you can't crank it up any more, pinch your thumbnail against your middle finger pad and take a deep breath. Smile. That's it. Let go, breathe out, and relax!

o OK, this one's a bit different. This time you're going to remember a time where you got the giggles—something was just so funny. Maybe it was inappropriate and you just couldn't stop laughing. And if you can't remember such a time, imagine if you could … even just a chuckle will do! Think of something you were completely amused by. Better still, think of something that made you laugh inside out.

Go on … have a go here. Remember what you saw in front of you at the time and make the images bigger, brighter, and more vivid. Make them appear all around you in 3D so they're completely real. Go on, crank it up! Remember what you heard at the time. Make it completely real so you can *feel* the sounds all around you. You're laughing in this scene. You just can't stop giggling, smiling, and laughing. It's like re-living it all over again. Remember all the other details and all the sensations you felt or could feel when you can't stop laughing.

Remember, you should be having fun with this. It's a key part of the formula, so go for it. Remember that funny time and re-live it now! Go on, really intensify all your senses, the sights, sounds, and feelings. Multiply everything by one hundred, and just when you can't crank it up any more, pinch your thumbnail against your middle finger pad and take a deep breath. Smile. That's it … and let go, breathe out, and relax!

o Well done, but just before we move onto the next part of the technique, let's just do one more of these. This time, you're going to recall all three intense states—confidence, curiosity, and hilarity—all at the same time! That's right, start with confidence. Remember how it felt to feel so confident. You knew you were going to do what it was with complete confidence and certainty. You can feel that right now. Remember what you were seeing and hearing. Remember how it feels right now. Take a deep breath and pinch your thumbnail against your middle finger. And now add that curiosity. Go on, mix them together … curiosity and confidence both together now. Remember what you saw and heard when you were feeling so curious right now, and mix that in with this amazing confidence. That's right. Keep it going, bigger and bigger, louder and more resonant. Literally feel your body vibrating with energy. Enjoy it, and pinch that thumbnail against your middle finger again. Really crank up these great feelings! And now add that laughter in. Mix it in with the confidence and the curiosity. Remember that time when maybe you shouldn't have been laughing but you couldn't stop yourself laughing. You're at least smiling right now. Remember what you saw and heard, make the images bigger, crisper, in 3D, and do the same with the sounds. Make them more resonant and louder and more real. Keep it up. Feel yourself smiling and even giggling. That's right, mix it in with the other wonderful states. Take a deep breath in, pinch that thumbnail against your middle finger … big smile … and relax!

Wow! How do you feel now?! You should feel very relaxed, possibly buzzed, and exhilarated. This is the first step. Now let's proceed to the next.

Step 2—The Old Movie Theater (two minutes)

This step is very straightforward. Simply read the instructions here and then close your eyes and follow the procedure in your mind. It will only take a minute or so.

Imagine you're sitting in a big movie theater. You're sitting right in the middle at ground floor level, and you're looking at an old sepia/black-and-white screen. It's old, and the movie you're going to watch is all crackly.

So, you're sitting there looking up at the cinema screen. And here's what you see: you're watching an old movie of the last time you had an episode where you became anxious and had the negative, destructive thought patterns running through your mind. If there's anything in particular that bothers or frustrates you, particularly anything that might adversely affect your health, you can include that context in this scenario.

So, just to recap, you're watching an old black-and-white movie, in normal speed, of the last time you had the negative thought pattern cycling in your mind. Get to the end of the movie safely and then open your eyes again. This process should take anything from twenty second to a minute.

Step 3—Disassociation and Rewind (five to ten minutes)

Here's where the magic happens. This is where you disassociate from the problem issue and then we rewind the movie you've just played, over and over again, until the negative feelings and by-products are literally erased.

Again, read these instructions and then close your eyes and follow the procedure.

OK, so there you are, imagining yourself sitting in that movie theater, having just watched the old crackly black-and-white movie of yourself having an episode, and that old movie is now paused at the very end of it.

Now imagine that you're floating up and back out of your body, watching the back of yourself sitting in the movie theater. Keep floating up and back right to the top and back of the movie theater. Open the door to the projection booth and enter inside, closing the door behind you; hear it click shut. You're now completely safe and secure, inside the projection booth, observing yourself down in the theater looking up at the old black-and-white movie screen.

Now play the movie backward. Now do it again. And again, this time faster. And another time. Each time you rewind it, rewind the movie faster, and as soon as it's rewound, do it again. You're in the projection booth, looking down at yourself in the cinema, looking up at the old movie screen, rewinding that black-and-white movie of yourself, faster and faster.

Take a deep breath, keep rewinding that movie, and pinch your thumbnail against your middle finger. Feel that confidence, curiosity, and laughter coursing through you as you breathe deeply and smile—and keep rewinding that movie. Go on, rewind it again and again and again! Now you're rewinding so fast each rewind blurs into the next.

Take another deep breath … and relax!

How do you feel? Think about those issues that bugged you before, and consider how you now feel about them. Are they winding you up so much anymore?

Gather yourself and repeat the above process again.

Again, you're inside the projection booth, observing yourself down in the theater looking up at the old black-and-white movie screen.

Play the movie backward. Do it again. And again, faster and faster. And another time. Each time you rewind it, rewind the movie faster, and as soon as it's rewound, do it again. You're in the projection booth,

71

looking down at yourself in the cinema, looking up at the old movie screen, rewinding that black-and-white movie of yourself, faster and faster.

Take a deep breath, keep rewinding that movie, and pinch your thumbnail against your middle finger. Feel that confidence, curiosity, and laughter as you breathe deeply and smile—and keep rewinding that movie. Go on, rewind it again and again and again! You're rewinding so fast each rewind blurs into the next.

For extra effect, when you do the rewinds, imagine everyone moving like the old movies, everyone in the movie speaking backward with helium voices, and try to imagine the silliest soundtrack for the rewind—something like the Benny Hill music. Make yourself laugh with this if you can, while still encouraging the positive states of confidence, curiosity, and laughter all at the same time. The more ridiculous you make it the better, and the more effective the technique will work. Really go for it and have fun! If you find yourself laughing, then so much the better, but it will be effective even if you don't laugh, so don't worry!

This entire process takes no more than twenty minutes and is truly remarkable. The old thinking pattern is either eliminated or at least greatly disempowered. Monitor yourself over the next few days. Your thinking will be clearer, calmer, and more peaceful—and your gut. Witness the transformation for yourself.

If you do nothing else in this book, do this! This is the most powerful technique I have ever found, and it works. You owe it to yourself to do it. If you want someone to help you with it, you can go to the www.yourgutfeeling.com website where you can download all my audio files for less than the price of one counseling session with a New York therapist. It is so worth it. Alternatively, you can find yourself a hypnotherapist or NLP practitioner who knows how to do the "Fast

Phobia Cure" or the "Rewind Technique." You'll need to show them this section of the book so they understand the context of what we're doing.

The main thing is that you understand how effective this process is, as implausible as it may sound. It is, in fact, a brilliant process that repairs the faulty wiring that has caused bad thinking habits. I have found the knock-on effect to be an immediate and remarkable calming down of the physical symptoms within a day or two.

Other Treatments and Therapies

These may be of assistance to you, but they weren't part of my recovery per se

o **Acupuncture**. This didn't do anything for me at the time, but in retrospect, I can say that it certainly shouldn't do any harm and could nicely supplement the hypnotherapy, because it will help you to relax.

o **Diets**. As you've read, they weren't core to my recovery. However, use your common sense and listen to your body. Don't eat anything that may have an aggravating effect on you personally. Get yourself tested for allergies, sure. But once you've done all that, if you're not improving noticeably, then you'll need to think out of the box a bit and then consider what I did.

Do listen to your body with all these things. Notice the effect of something like drinking coffee. After having no coffee for almost a year, my first cup sent me straight to the ceiling … and the bathroom too! It wasn't a problem, but caffeine is a known laxative, even more so if you're not used to it. Now I'll drink anything I like, but I can notice the difference that caffeine has on me. Similarly, be aware of the effect of different foods on you in general. Too much sugar can send people to sleep. These are effects outside of the conditions in question here, but it's a smart thing to be aware of how food and drink affects you in general ... without being an obsessive bore about them! There's a difference between awareness and fanaticism!

I was enthusiastic about every treatment until I'd given it a chance. With some things I gave them too much of a chance. But soon after I started Geoffrey's treatment, it was clear that something big was changing. It was subtle at first, but listening to my body, something was happening that hadn't happened after any of the other things that I'd been trying.

As an aside, for your next step after you've dealt with the mind side of things, for increased energy and overall wellbeing, you may want to consider a more "Alkaline" lifestyle. This is a common-sense approach based on over 30 years of research. The idea is to feed yourself with foods that work with your natural processes, leading to increased energy and vitality.

o **Herbs and Natural Remedies**. In terms of the colitis I believe certain herbs and natural remedies won't do you any harm and may even have a placebo effect. If so, great. But I do believe their effect could be moderate at best because they do seem to avoid the main issue, which isn't necessarily physical in the first place.

I used some of the Nature's Sunshine products for a time. When I stopped using them, there wasn't the slightest difference in my condition, but for a while after being well they represented my physical effort and contribution to treating that part of my body with respect. My view was that that part of my body had suffered, and therefore I was going to give it the best nutrients to continue the good work I'd already done with

Geoffrey. Chronologically, it's important to understand that I was already making giant strides in my recovery before I started using these products.

This is not a plug for Nature's Sunshine, and I have no association with them whatsoever. I'm purely repeating what I did here for what it's worth. The ones I did use were:

➔ Bowel Detox (formerly Bowel Build)

➔ Intestinal Soothe & Build (formerly UC3-J), a blend of herbs

➔ Slippery Elm Bark

➔ Capsicum—this is basically red chili (cayenne) pepper. It's very hot (spicy) and has healing properties.

All the above come in capsules, so you won't have to actually taste them. Frankly you wouldn't want to taste them!

As an aside, once I was fully well again, I started taking a fiber supplement and still do to this day. My rationale was that I may as well keep things ticking over down there, and from day to day I simply wanted to ensure I was getting enough fiber in my diet. When I was ill, I was desperate to stop the moving, so this was only a factor when I was fully recovered. My view was that I could sustain my recovery with both Geoffrey's techniques, reinforced with simply being sensible. But remember, I eat what I want when I want and have no restrictions whatsoever.

o   More latterly, I've also found energy benefits in simple good nutrition and making sure I'm ingesting more "Alkaline" produce. This is purely for more energy and wellbeing, which I'm sure you'll agree is a good thing! You can find more details on www.yourgutfeeling.com/energise.

o **Exercise**. This actually played no role in my recovery, but I'm adding it in here anyway. The reason is that if you can exercise, it's a wonderful thing. When I was ill, I didn't dare for obvious reasons. At school I was always a team sports player, but nowadays I love to swim about a mile whenever possible. Swimming is a unique exercise that can have amazing benefits to your mental state. Here's why.

First, when you swim you are weightless. Second, your body motion is (or should be!) smooth and circular. Third, if you swim *properly*, then you'll learn how to breathe when you're in the water. Trust me, it's incredible how that makes you feel after thirty minutes; endorphins galore! And finally, it's just a great de-stressor from the point of view that it's a great work out. The secret is to have swimming lessons so you know how to breathe while you're in the water, and so you know how to move properly while you're in it. In summary, swimming is amazing therapy.

Summary

What I did was not rocket science. It was all underpinned by my attitude and fighting spirit. That enabled me to keep looking until I succeeded. My attitude included being open-minded. All that mattered was the end result, and I really didn't care how I got there. I think that sitting on a chair and being spoken to nicely is a pretty good way of making a recovery! But that belies the extraordinary science that is behind proper treatment.

If for any reason you had reservations about hypnosis before reading this book, how do you feel about it now? How do you feel about the rewind technique? How important is it for you to be completely well again? Are you willing to give it a proper try? For me it was a no-brainer. If being well is your priority, then you'll find the right person to help you and you'll give it a try.

If things in this book have resonated with you, then you owe it to yourself to start believing you can be well and now start acting on it. The healthy state is the natural state, and you're entitled to be healthy, provided you're not abusing it every day! I'm not looking for you to be a health freak. Let's just lead a normal, healthy life with no restrictions, just like most others. That's the attitude. Now, go and do it yourself.

Hypnotic Induction and Suggestions

What now follows is a transcript of Geoffrey's hypnotic induction and the actual words that he used with me. In the right-hand column I explain how elements of the trance work.

The reason for this is so you can understand and appreciate the structure of this skill and underpin your belief in its effectiveness. It's not essential that you understand how or why it works, but it is important that you believe in the power of this method and in your ability to replicate it for your own benefit.

To download this recording and the other bonus relaxation recording, go to www.yourgutfeeling.com.

Geoffrey Glassborow's Hypnotic Induction

Now get yourself completely comfortable. Close your eyes and keep them firmly shut until I tell you to open them.

Other methods such as pendulums can also be used for the initial part.

Now think of your breathing. Breathe more deeply than normal. Deep, steady breathing, deep and steady, deep steady breathing and keep that up. As you breathe in this way, feel the relaxation flowing throughout your body. Relax. Breathe deeply, steadily, and relax, deep, steady, and relax, and let go.

Notice the importance of breathing, right at the beginning of the induction. Deep, steady breathing helps the process of going into trance.

Now think of different parts of your body, starting with your feet, your right foot, the muscles relaxing the joints going limp and the tension going, your left foot, the muscles relaxing the joints going limp and the tension going, your right hand, the muscles relaxing the joints going limp and the tension going, your left hand, the muscles relaxing the joints going limp and the tension going, your right leg, the muscles relaxing the joints going limp and the tension going, your left leg, the muscles relaxing the joints going limp and the tension going, your right arm, the muscles relaxing the joints going limp and the tension going, your left arm, the muscles relaxing the joints going limp and the tension going, your feet and hands and legs and arms becoming more an more relaxed and still and tranquil and peaceful, peace and inner calm spreading throughout your body toward your brain.

Notice the use of repetition and rhythm.

With the breathing deep and steady, now we're going on a journey around the body, literally instructing it to start relaxing all over.

Feel the drowsiness deepening gradually toward that halfway stage between wakefulness and sleep, the twilight state. And remember, this is a joint effort between the two of us, it's a partnership . We are creating a great force, a force that will last, continue to help you indefinitely, the partnership continues.

Now the whole of the trunk of your body the muscles and fibers relaxing, the spine going limp and the tension going, and your neck, the muscles relaxing and the vertebrae going limp and the tension going, the base of your skull, the nerves relaxing, helping the nervous system throughout the rest of your body relax still further. The back of your head and ears relaxing and the tension going, the top of your head relaxing and the tension going, and your face relaxing and the tension going, your mouth, all the muscles of your mouth relaxing and your chin, the muscles relaxing and your tongue, the muscles relaxing and your throat the muscles relaxing.

Your breathing easy, relaxed, steady, controlled, and deeper. As you breathe out, breathe out the tension from the innermost corners of your body, as you breathe in breathe in the relaxation that will replace that tension. Fill your body with relaxation and goodness.

Notice the reference to partnership. We can form a similar partnership by way of this book and the recordings.

More references to the body and instructing it to relax. This part is quite lengthy because we knew it was being recorded for when I was going away. In a live, non-recorded session, we would often skip this part because I'd be "under" very quickly anyway.

A reminder as to the breathing. "Easy, steady, controlled, and deeper." "Easy" being the most important here.

Feel the growing warmth and coziness, relaxation and drowsiness, stillness and tranquility, peace and detachment, inner calm, a drift toward a deeper state … which you're going to achieve, I'm going to help you achieve.

I'm going to count to twenty, and as I do so, I want you to encourage the feeling of deepening relaxation, and as I count, I put my hand on your forehead … feel the help and strength coming across through this contact.

Feel this as a very real physical force going right through you like a charge of electricity. Feel a slight warmth of my fingertips, a tingling sensation, and let go toward a deeper (sensation of) relaxation, a deeper drowsiness, the twilight state as I count.

One, two, three, four, five, six, seven, eight, nine, ten, eleven, twelve, thirteen, fourteen, fifteen, sixteen, seventeen eighteen, nineteen, twenty.

And now use your imagination. Imagine that you're becoming very, very light, so light that you begin to float. Even though your reason tells you you're not, imagine that you are. Think of yourself floating, feel yourself floating, sense yourself floating, see yourself floating. Picture it, floating, and as you float there's a slight swaying sensation, swaying and drifting, floating, swaying, and drifting, the relaxation getting deeper and a feeling of great inner peace and calm and tranquility growing. And a drowsiness and a sleepiness coming over you, but still aware. Drowsy and sleepy, drowsy and sleepy, but aware.

Part of the hypnotic phenomenon is that you do not have to say things with perfect grammar. In fact, it's often best to use deliberately confusing or ambiguous language that isn't grammatically correct.

Notice the laying of hands on my forehead. This is very much part of Geoffrey's method yet it still worked even when I simply listened to the tape for two months. The suggestion of the physical contact is

Take note of the rhythm of what is being said here and the metronome in the background adding another dimension to sound as well as setting a beat for the breathing. powerful even without the actual contact itself

And now concentrate on your right arm, that too becoming incredibly light, even lighter than the rest of you, and your right arm will float upward, and you will feel it, feel the lightness of your right hand and arm, light and floating, floating in air, floating … upward. Feel it, feel the wonderful sensation of this incredible lightness and floating, wonderful. And all the time it floats, you're getting rid of all the negative forces from yourself and your inner self, getting rid of the tension and the anxiety, the depression, getting rid of all the doubts and fears and self doubts, getting rid of all the negative forces and negative thoughts and negative emotions. Getting rid of the physical problem, the colitis, getting rid of everything that stands between you and the quality of life that you're looking for. Feel it. Getting rid of all those negative forces, feel the relief.

And now look in your mind at a picture of yourself. You see completely new life spreading before you, you're free, free from the physical restraints of the past, totally fit, very successful in your career, bags of energy to do more and more, very successful in your emotional and home life, looking very, very happy. You see a totally relaxed person, and because of this relaxed state, you always have great energy and alertness and creativity and drive and enthusiasm and determination and the will to succeed and absolute control at all times. You're completely healthy in body and mind. You sleep perfectly every night, waking fully refreshed every morning, full of confidence in yourself and confidence in the present and confidence in the future and confidence in your ability to achieve whatever you wish. You think positively, you enjoy life when you can; you make the best of things when you have to. You have a feeling of wellbeing. All is well with you, the feeling of wellbeing that comes from the state of relaxation, confidence, and control, and through these three forces you see yourself transformed.

Sometimes my arm would drift, sometimes it wouldn't, and sometimes I was already out by now! It actually doesn't matter. All that matters is that you're getting nicely relaxed by now and at least being able to *imagine* the arm floating. Being distracted on the arm enables the positive suggestions for other parts of the anatomy to be accepted.

We're now into the main body of the suggestions. By this time we're nicely relaxed and able to use our imagination whilst in a highly suggestible state.

Relaxation, confidence, and control, remember these three words always, remember to repeat them to yourself at least once a day, and as you repeat them, think of the meaning of the words and how they apply to your particular situations. Relaxation, confidence, and control. Remember also that you can do anything you want, anything at all, provided it's within your capabilities, you can do anything you want. Your capabilities are far greater than you imagine them to be. This gives you all the scope you need. You can do anything.

That means also that you can be involved in getting rid of the colitis or any other physical problem that you encounter because you can do anything you want, you can achieve total fitness by your own efforts, and it is right that you should see this and believe it.

I'm going to put my hand on your forehead again, and I want you to put your hands over the area that has been causing the problem, the area of the bowel. Now I want you to concentrate all your thoughts on that particular area. Feel a growing warmth coming to it and healing. [*period of silence*] Feel it. And picture all the healing forces of your body gathering together, moving toward this area in little armies and cleaning it. All the healing forces now descending on that area that has caused the problem, the inflammation, and healing it, getting rid of the inflammation, and you can feel that with your hands, you can feel it in progress, slowly but surely … it is working, and you can keep it working until you're totally, absolutely fit.

Notice the reference to real life here. "You enjoy life when you can; you make the best of things when you have to." This is very much part of Geoffrey's no-nonsense, realistic approach to his work. What he's saying here is life will have its ups and downs and you'll be able to cope during those down times.

Relaxation, confidence, and control. These are the three lynchpins upon Geoffrey's approach. If you're relaxed, then this has great benefits to your entire body and mental state. If you're confident ,then you can move forward in life without hesitation. If you're in control, then you will control your thoughts and actions. The implication of this is that you can also be in control of your physical state.

Now you can let the healing forces return to their respective areas, where they will settle down and await the next demand. Turn your own hands to the arm of the chair. I take my hands off your forehead and feel, feel the benefit of healing, of healing yourself.

And now I'm going to count from ten to one, and as I count, you'll feel lighter and lighter, and when I reach one, you'll open you eyes. You'll then be fully aware and full of energy.

Ten, nine, eight, seven, six, five, four, three, two, one.

At this point I started to imagine fire trucks and fire-fighters as the "armies" inside my body, clearing up the damage and hosing away the nastiness with powerful jets of ice-cool water, cooling everything down, like water putting out some burning embers. There's something innately good about fire-fighters and this concept of cooling things down. I'd also imagine the water cleaning up the pipes as it were. From rusty and unhealthy to sparkling and shiny. You can use whatever imagery you like, but these worked for me.

Notice also the words "feel the benefit … of healing yourself." This puts the privilege firmly onto you, meaning you can self-perpetuate the virtuous cycle that has been started here. Effectively, what he's saying here is that you're in charge and you now have the ability to continue the good work.

Interview with Geoffrey Glassborow

Guy: Well, Geoffers, this was quite a journey, wasn't it!

Geoffrey: It certainly was. Job well done, I'd say!

Guy: Let's just explain for the benefit of the listeners here. We met in June 1995, after I'd been ill for about a year.

Geoffrey: That is correct.

Guy: When I met you, I was twenty-four years old, nine stone in weight (around 126 pounds or 58 kilos), and in pretty bad shape. You were seventy-three years old, hugely experienced as a hypnotherapist, and you knew you could help my particular situation. It's also worth noting that you knew our family, not so much me, but you knew my parents already.

So, as I remember it, I could have been just a bit tetchy when we first met, wouldn't you say?!

Geoffrey: Well, that's an understatement! But you were very ill at the time, so it wasn't a surprise. But I'm used to seeing people like that when they meet me for the first time. Your particular problem was borne out of bad thinking, as it is with many sufferers. The difference with you was that you were open to this concept from the very beginning. I had no battles with you in that sense. Many people can be highly resistant to change, even if they've got themselves into a real mess. You simply wanted to get better, which made things slightly easier for me!

Guy: I remember very clearly, you asking me in that first session what I wanted to achieve, and I said, "A complete recovery" before going into minute detail about what that meant. And you kept saying that if I just concentrated on being totally fit and healthy that would cover all bases and I didn't need to obsess about the details.

Geoffrey: Well, that's right. If you're totally fit, then by definition you couldn't be ill in any way. It's then a question of using your imagination vividly but in a constructive way. It's not about what you're *not* going to have, as you were expressing it, but more the vitality of what you *are* going to have that will propel you toward healthiness.

Guy: I noticed that very quickly; that, in effect, you were teaching me how to think ... or at least teaching me how to think *properly*.

Geoffrey: Well, yes. Most people don't consciously notice how they communicate internally with themselves. Many people, like you, get into bad thinking habits that cause exaggerated stress, which then can lead to physical symptoms. In your case, and many others I've seen over the years, that was precisely the case.

With stomach problems people would be astonished how much can be resolved by attacking the problem in a different way—I mean, through the mind. I've seen cases of IBS, Crohn's, and colitis, and in many cases there were obvious common denominators.

Guy: Such as?

Geoffrey: Well, first I can hear tension in someone's voice and the speed at which they speak—it's a tell-tale sign. I pay attention to their breathing, which is often very shallow. I remember you said at the time that you could barely breathe. Well, that's a sign of tension and the chest cavity not being relaxed. If the stomach is uncomfortable, then that in itself makes breathing properly more difficult, so it can become a vicious circle.

Other major factors are relationships, either with partners or family, parents, or siblings, which has contributed to the long-term bad thinking habits in the first place.

So, there are a few things that are instantly recognizable in people with these problems, but the next challenge is to get them to recognize what the issues are voluntarily, and then how to become healthy with or without those other issues still in the background.

Guy: So, the underlying root cause doesn't necessarily have to be fixed or confronted?

Geoffrey: Only internally. There's no point in trying to fix other people around you or how they behave; that's never going to be productive. It's a question of changing your own interpretation of their behavior and how you react to it. I guess you can always get away from those people, but then you still have to deal with the bad thinking habits that have accumulated over the years. So, you do address the issue, but you do so in a clever way. Besides, I'm not there to interfere with anyone's personal relationships. With the right armory you can do that for yourself. My job is to give you the armory to be strong.

Guy: What are the typical bad thinking habits?

Geoffrey: They typically manifest themselves in self-argument. In other words, people literally go around and have arguments in their minds either with themselves or people like their parents.

Guy: I can relate to having imaginary arguments in my mind. I did it constantly. I even remember a lunch break where I went to get my sandwiches and was actively looking forward to walking in the park and having a good old argument in my mind!

Geoffrey: That's exactly it. It's a typical sign of serious insecurity, and if it gets out of hand, it can lead to physical problems, just like in your case.

Guy: So how do we stop the spiral of decline?

Geoffrey: Well, it's partly a matter of learning how to *think* properly. We do this from a couple of angles but always trying to keep things as simple as possible.

So, for a start, when we chat, before the hypnosis, I'm influencing the structure of your thinking. Just like I did when I asked you what your goal was. You were fixated on the detail, and I got you to concentrate on overall fitness, not the detail of the illness and how those details would be fixed.

For everyday thinking, and to assist your ongoing health, I make you aware of those destructive inner voice arguments. Once you're aware of them, you can start to question them and eliminate them. Once you eliminate the noise inside your mind, then you can begin to relax. Once you can relax, the more productive you can be, and the better you will feel.

I also teach you how to breathe, not just from a hypnotic point of view, but also for every day. So now you're thinking more healthily and you're breathing properly. Just those small changes alone go a long way to easing the intestinal condition. But there's a lot more that's going on behind the scenes. That's where the hypnosis comes in.

During hypnosis you learn how to get into a relaxed state. Once you're in it, then my suggestions will reinforce what we discuss outside of the trance. So you now have conscious learning with unconscious understanding and reinforcement. I also emphasize the power of partnership. I become partners with all my clients. The power of two people is more than double the power of one person. And somehow, this mix turns out to be profoundly powerful with a range of intestinal and skin (dermis) disorders, as well as a number of other conditions.

Guy: Is it the same for everyone?

Geoffrey: Well, of course nothing's identical for any two people, but there are a lot of common denominators that in this sort of thing seem to get the right results. But the key thing is always the individual themselves. I have a basic structure that I tailor and adapt for each individual, but the structure is very much there.

Because you were so determined and so open to learning and changing in order to get well, you did get well, and you did it quite quickly.

Guy: Well, we negotiated, didn't we! Do you remember, during that first session you said, "Well, a day is too soon … but a year is too long …" and we went back and forth until we settled on six months. And sure enough, six months later the same doctors that had been urging me to have surgery and saying I'd never be well were pronouncing that I may as well forget I'd ever been ill in the first place!

Geoffrey: Well, yes … and you have to take credit for that.

Guy: Sure, but it also only happened because you'd given me the mechanisms and techniques. I was about to get married at the time, and I listened to your tape when I was away before the wedding and on the honeymoon. And you know what, I made giant strides in that month that I was away, just listening to your tape. That's why I' thought we should include it here.

Geoffrey: Yes, well, there wouldn't be any point in re-recording something that had such a great effect.

Guy: Definitely not. And I think that it's even more powerful that this is *the* recording that did it for me even when I was away. It wouldn't have been the same if it was made purposely for being a recording. This one somehow has real physical presence.

Geoffrey: Absolutely, and that's for anyone who listens to it.

Guy: So Geoffers, what's your advice for people who are suffering from IBS, Crohn's, or colitis?

Geoffrey: Well, now that this book has been written, they should read it for sure. It's not often that a real-life case study becomes so accessible and with these types of conditions very few people are willing to discuss the symptoms. As you said, many people feel a lack of dignity, and that's not easy to talk about, even years later. Also, not many people have your experience of making a full recovery from it.

You really need to be honest with yourself and then be logical. Is there any point in being treated exclusively by someone who doesn't believe they can help you get well? That just doesn't make sense, does it?

From there, it's about determination, technique, and perhaps a bit of luck. But you rarely get the luck without the determination, so in these types of cases, you make your own luck.

Guy: Geoffrey, I know people who won't go near hypnosis. They think it's either going to manipulate them or they don't want someone "prying" into their innermost thoughts. All the usual objections. What do you say to those people?

Geoffrey: The fear of hypnosis is typically borne out of ignorance, misrepresentation, or the odd story about an unethical practitioner. The stage hypnotist shows are a two-edged sword. On the one hand they bring awareness of hypnosis, but on the other, they can be misleading. From a therapeutic point of view, the stage hypnosis may as well be a totally different practice altogether. In hypnotherapy, we're a team. We cooperate, and nothing is done without the express agreement of the patient and therapist.

Look how many people have benefited from hypnosis. Look how many smokers become non-smokers. Phobias are melted away; pain is numbed; people like you have been cured from "incurable" illnesses. How can you argue with that? Surely, it's worth a shot on that basis alone … if you really want to make the change. And even if it's a last resort, and typically it is, who wouldn't want to give themselves at least a fighting chance of accomplishing the challenge in question, whatever that might be? But, some people will always have their suspicions, no matter what the evidence.

Guy: And what do you say to them?

Geoffrey: Well, if someone is that suspicious about hypnotherapy, then at least they believe it has some effect. So if they're suspicious it could be used for bad, it means they must also believe it can be used for good. From there, it's just a matter of finding someone you feel comfortable with and can trust. Also, talk with people who've had it done for any other problem and find out what they thought.

Guy: Like I said, I was almost disappointed that I wasn't sleep-walking by the end! In fact, in our first several sessions I was awake, albeit very relaxed. I knew exactly what you'd said. Nowadays I'd just let go completely and probably fall asleep.

Geoffrey: And the great thing is that it doesn't actually matter if you weren't asleep. The main point is that it worked.

Guy: It certainly did … and that's a good place to leave this interview. Many thanks, Geoffers.

Geoffrey: And thanks to you, Guy. This is a real pleasure, and this project is going to help a lot of people.

Appendix

Official Definitions

This section is more about defining IBD conditions in more detail. Descriptions are taken from journals and other references, so I apologize if much of what follows is written in a more clinical and formal style. Interestingly, they all refer to stress in a rather glib way as having an effect on these conditions. What I've done in the previous sections is to define exactly what we mean by stress (i.e., bad thinking) and what we can do to get rid of it regardless of life's ups and downs.

Even now, I'm slightly bemused by the fact that the reference to "stress" is so matter of fact and unexplored. So, this section is for your background general knowledge more than anything else. Frankly, it's optional.

IBS

Irritable bowel syndrome (IBS) is a common disorder of the intestines that leads to cramps, abdominal pain, flatulence, bloating, and changes in bowel habits. Some people with IBS have constipation; others have diarrhea, often with great urgency; and some people experience both. Sometimes the person with IBS suffers with painful cramps together with an urge to move the bowels but cannot do so.

IBS has been referred to by many names: colitis, mucous colitis, spastic colon, spastic bowel, and functional bowel disease. Most of these terms are technically inaccurate from a clinical perspective. For example, colitis refers specifically to inflammation of the large intestine (colon). IBS, however, does not involve inflammation. Therefore, although we are going to tackle them in the same way here, they are, clinically at least, distinct conditions. In strict medical terms, IBS is not yet considered a disease but a syndrome or collection of symptoms. I emphasize the word yet! Conditions such as colitis are often accompanied with IBS symptoms.

The cause of IBS is not known, and as yet there is no clinical cure per se. In other words, there is no cure that has been found treating the condition by way of drugs. I was told the same thing with ulcerative colitis, yet I've been free from it for over nine years … and counting. Doctors call IBS a functional disorder because there is no sign of disease when the colon is examined.

IBS causes a great deal of discomfort and distress, but it does not physically cause permanent harm to the intestines and does not lead to intestinal bleeding of the bowel or other diseases. IBS can range from a mild annoyance to something seriously disabling. Those afflicted may be unable to go to social events, to go out to a job, or to travel even short distances. Many people with IBS, however, are able to exercise some control over their symptoms through prescription medications, diet, and relaxation techniques.

Causes of IBS

The colon, which is about six feet long, connects the small intestine with the rectum and anus. The major function of the colon is to absorb water and salts from digestive products that enter from the small intestine. Two quarts of liquid matter enter the colon from the small intestine each day. This material may remain there for several days until most of the fluid and salts are absorbed into the body. The stool then passes through the colon by a pattern of movements to the left side of the colon, where it is stored until a bowel movement occurs.

Colon motility (contraction of intestinal muscles and movement of its contents) is controlled by nerves and hormones and by electrical activity in the colon muscle. The electrical activity is thought to as a pacemaker similar to the mechanism that controls heart function.

Movements of the colon propel the contents slowly back and forth but mainly toward the rectum. A few times each day strong muscle contractions move down the colon, pushing fecal material ahead of them. Some of these strong contractions result in a bowel movement.

Because doctors have been unable to find an organic cause, IBS often has been thought to be caused by emotional conflict or stress. Stress can considerably worsen IBS symptoms, and research suggests that the colon muscle of a person with IBS begins to spasm after only mild stimulation. The person with IBS seems to have a colon that is more sensitive and reactive than usual, so it responds strongly to stimuli that would not bother most people.

Ordinary events, such as eating and distention from gas or other material in the colon, can cause the colon to overreact in the person with IBS. Certain medicines and foods can trigger spasms in some people. Sometimes the spasm delays the passage of stool, leading to constipation. Chocolate, milk products, or large amounts of alcohol are thought to be frequent offenders, but not in all sufferers. Caffeine can cause loose stools in many people, but it is more likely to affect those with IBS. Researchers also have found that women with IBS can have more symptoms during their menstrual periods, suggesting that reproductive hormones can increase IBS symptoms. Again, notice the common link of stress.

The first symptoms of IBS often appear in a person's late teens or twenties. IBS tends to diminish in severity with age, but millions of elderly people also have it.

Though it's not clear why, IBS is most prevalent among Caucasians, affecting more women than men. Approximately 67 percent of IBS sufferers are female. No conclusive reasons have been identified, other than emotional issues or past traumas. Again, this reinforces the theme of this book, as the gastrointestinal tract is extremely sensitive to stress.

Diet and Stress

Note that diet played no part in my recovery, so I'm skeptical about it in this context.

The potential for abnormal function of the colon is present in people with IBS, but it is thought that a trigger must also be present to cause symptoms. The most likely culprits seem to be diet and emotional stress. Many people report that their symptoms occur following a meal or when they are under stress. No one is sure why this happens, but scientists think they have some clues. Unfortunately, these clues haven't led them to any effective treatments.

Stress also stimulates colonic spasm in people with IBS. This process is not completely understood, but scientists point out that the colon is controlled partly by the nervous system. Stress reduction through relaxation training can help relieve IBS symptoms. In my language, this means learning how to think more healthily in a relaxed state.

Look at what I have been through. It's not the normal ebb and flow of life that affects the gut. It's the way we handle ourselves through those peaks and troughs that's so important. That's what my story is all about. I've been through much more stress as a well person than I ever did when I was ill.

Links to Other Conditions

IBS has not been shown to lead to any serious, organic diseases. It is alleged that no link has been established between IBS and inflammatory bowel diseases such as Crohn's disease or ulcerative colitis. However, IBS inherently goes with those other conditions too, so how can there be no link? Also, the types of stress that accompany all these conditions have strong common denominators. I'm all for measuring things so double-blind studies can be performed. However, measurements need to be qualitative as well as quantitative, particularly when drug therapies and traditional medicine have such a poor record of treatment for these types of conditions.

Diagnosis

IBS usually is diagnosed after doctors exclude the presence of disease. To get to that point, the doctor will take a complete medical history that includes a careful description of symptoms and drug history, because many drugs can causes abdominal distress and other IBS symptoms. A physical examination and laboratory tests will be done. A stool sample will be tested for evidence of bleeding. The doctor also may do diagnostic procedures such as X-rays or endoscopy (viewing the colon through a flexible tube inserted through the anus) to find out if there is disease.

It may be sensible to review your travel over the past year with your doctor, especially trips to third-world countries abroad. It's possible that you picked up an intestinal bug, and your doctor can carry out tests as such. Again, this is more for ruling out other things.

Undiagnosed diabetes can cause symptoms of IBS. Your doctor might ask you to take a glucose-tolerance test and a blood test for diabetes. Other tests can be taken to rule out ulcers, intestinal polyps, diverticular disease, pancreatitis, colitis, Crohn's disease, an intestinal blockage, and other diseases.

IBS Warning Signs

It is thought that IBS rarely progresses to more severe conditions. However, in my case, I certainly had the IBS part well before the bleeding set in. So again, I'm not sure about this theory. My concern about so many of these theories is that they don't lead to anything constructive. What I did does lead to something constructive, and that's what you need.

IBS symptoms may vary over time, and some symptoms warrant professional attention. Specialist consultation is recommended if you experience any of these symptoms or situations:

- **Fever**. If you develop a fever in addition to your abdominal symptoms, it suggests something else is present, like a bacteria, bug, or even appendicitis.
- **Vomiting**. If you begin vomiting in addition to your abdominal symptoms, it suggests an infection or even an ulcer.
- **Black or bloody stools**. These suggest gastrointestinal bleeding, a possible sign of an ulcer, colitis, or Crohn's disease.
- **Persistent abdominal pain**. Persistent pain or pain that comes and goes after eating could mean an ulcer, gallstones, diverticular disease, or appendicitis.

- **Symptoms worsen**. If your symptoms suddenly become significantly worse, and the new symptoms persist for more than a few days, it might be a sign of any of the conditions already mentioned.
- **Persistent lower abdominal pain**. For women, this might be a sign of endometriosis, a uterine fibroid, or some other gynecological condition.
- **Unintended weight loss**. This could be anything really, but shouldn't be too much of a surprise because discomfort in the abdomen rarely leads to a big appetite.

Treatment

1. Lifestyle Changes

Lifestyle changes can make a difference in controlling symptoms. Also, there are a few over-the-counter and prescription medications that can help relieve some discomfort in some cases. These didn't work for me, but I certainly gave them a try. IBS is rarely curable in the same way as an infection. So traditionally, relief has come only from learning how to control its symptoms over time. Remember, I had much worse than this and would not accept control only. I wanted to be rid of the thing, and that's what I did.

Mainstream medicine and alternative therapies are geared toward the goal of controlling the condition, though certain lifestyle modifications are also thought to help.

- **Eat less fat**. A high-fat diet can contribute to heart disease, obesity, and other serious conditions. It is thought that it can aggravate IBS, too, though I can't verify this, certainly not in my experience of being ill. The emphasis here is "aggravate." Where IBS is not present, there is no evidence to suggest a high-fat diet could induce the condition.

- **Eat more fiber**. Fiber is the roughage in fruits, vegetables, beans, and whole-grain items. A high-fiber diet adds bulk to the stool and is a cornerstone of treating constipation. Many people find that it also helps control IBS, though some find it can aggravate it more. FiberSmart is a mild and safe fiber supplement.

- **Be cautious with wheat bran**. As you increase how much fiber you eat, pay attention to how wheat bran affects you. Researchers at the University Hospital of South Manchester in England surveyed one hundred people with IBS who were eating bran as a source of fiber. Ten percent reported improvement, but 55 percent said it made them worse. If bran aggravates your IBS, eliminate it and get fiber from other sources.

- **Avoid substances that irritate the gastrointestinal tract**. Anything that irritates the digestive tract can aggravate IBS. In addition to high-fat foods, bran, and lactose (if you're intolerant), common irritants include alcohol, caffeine, carbonated beverages, and the fruit-derived sweetener sorbitol. Nicotine can irritate the gastrointestinal tract, too, so if you smoke, here's another reason to quit.

- **Eat less sugar**. In one study, two groups ate the same diet for two weeks, except that one group ate an additional four ounces of sugar a day. In the sugar group, colonic peristalsis and intestinal gas formation both increased. These changes increase risk of IBS. Sugar is one of modern-day life's great problems for other reasons, so it's a good thing to try and wean yourself off anyway.

2. Drug Therapy

I'm all for trying anything, so by all means, try whatever you can and see if it makes a real difference to you.

There is no standard way of treating IBS. That's mainly because physicians simply don't understand the root cause of the condition. I believe that I do in the vast majority of cases, hence my approach in this course, which worked on me with a far worse condition. Remember, I tried all sorts things, many of which I haven't detailed here yet.

Your doctor may prescribe fiber supplements or occasional laxatives if you are constipated. Some doctors prescribe drugs that control colon muscle spasms, drugs that slow the movement of food through the digestive system, or tranquilizers, all of which may relieve symptoms. Antidepressant drugs also are used sometimes in patients who are depressed. Out of all these, I'd be more inclined to look at the antidepressants or tranquilizers, except for the fact that they can be highly addictive for certain types of personalities.

- **Antispasmodics**. If abdominal pain or cramping is a significant part of your IBS, antispasmodic medication may help ease the painful contractions of the muscles that surround the intestine. Dosages will vary with the particular drug and how it's formulated. If you have questions about dosage, talk with a pharmacist or your physician. Antispasmodics are safe for most people, but you should always check first, as they are not compatible for people with certain conditions, and they can, in cases, have side effects. I did try some of these during my first six months with colitis, though with no benefit.

- **Anti-diarrhea**. Anti-diarrhea medication is usually recommended only for occasional use, not for management of chronic conditions like IBS. However, your physician might recommend keeping antidiarrheals on hand, if diarrhea occasionally becomes severe and the non-drug treatment approaches don't provide enough relief. Immodium and Pepto Bismol are two medications I would always have in my cabinet anyway, and at times these can be highly effective at temporarily relieving symptoms. They are not, however, for continual day-in, day-out use, and you should at least get some supervision from a doctor with any medications.

- **Laxatives** Well, this was completely inappropriate for me—I couldn't stop going without the laxatives! For relief of constipation, laxatives are only for occasional use, not for the ongoing management of IBS. Your doctor may suggest that you keep some laxatives in your medicine cabinet, if constipation becomes severe from time to time and non-drug treatment doesn't give you enough relief. Having a consistent intake of fiber as a lifestyle may be helpful on an ongoing basis.

- **Bulk formers**. The most natural approach is to use bulk formers, which increase the size of stool. Bulkier stools press on the colon wall and stimulate the rectal muscle contractions that we experience as the urge to use the toilet. Dietary fiber is a bulk former, which is why a high-fiber diet is recommended for controlling IBS. A convenient way to take it is by using one of the many commercial packages that contain it (FiberSmart is natural, mild, and simply keeps things ticking over down there).

- **Lubricants**. I never tried these, but here's a description anyway. Mineral oil, a petroleum product, is the magic ingredient found in lubricant laxatives. These coat the stool to promote easier passage but shouldn't be used routinely. Over time, it depletes the body of fat-soluble vitamins (A, D, E, and K). And mineral oil may interfere with your body's ability to absorb other medications.

- **Saline laxatives**. Again, laxatives simply weren't what I needed. These change the salt balance in the digestive tract. They draw water into the stool, adding bulk and stimulating peristalsis. Milk of magnesia is the best-known saline laxative and shouldn't be used for extended periods. Always read the instructions and if in doubt, consult the pharmacist or doctor.

- **Stool softeners**. These also draw water into the stool, softening it and making it easier to pass. Drink plenty of nonalcoholic liquids with these products.

- **Chemical stimulants**. Stimulant laxatives can be unpleasantly powerful and are a last resort to stimulate rectal muscle contractions. They may cause cramping and bloody diarrhea. Using them for long periods can dependency on them.

- **Enemas**. Finally, some people use enemas to treat constipation. Enemas irrigate the bowel and act as lubricants and stimulants. But frequent enemas can damage the colon and cause electrolyte imbalances. As a result, doctors generally discourage them for this use.

  The enemas I was prescribed were steroid anti-inflammatories and sulphur-based—not for constipation. Once I realized that they weren't actually doing anything for my condition, I stopped using them. Again, by all means try different things, but do listen to your body. If there's no positive response, move onto something else until you find something that works. Drug treatments didn't work for me, but I only discovered that after going through the process of trying them.

- **Antidepressants and Tranquilizers**. Some studies have tested antidepressants as a treatment for IBS. Researchers analyzing the results of several such studies found that they all showed antidepressants to be more effective than placebos in treating abdominal pain and other gastrointestinal symptoms in some patients. Often the effective dosage was significantly less than it would be for treating depression.

  What do these results tell us? It really confirms what this book is all about—that IBS and these other conditions is more about the nervous system than anything else. Tranquilizers would also be useful on a strictly occasional basis if you need to take the edge off a particularly stressful episode. However, you do not want to take these regularly or become dependant. They would purely be used as a one-off.

3. Alternative Medicine in IBS

Very few who suffer from IBS find enough relief in mainstream medicine. Alternative medicine also offers a number of approaches with mixed results to control IBS symptoms.

- **Elimination diets**. Lactose intolerance is not the only food sensitivity that can cause or contribute to IBS type symptoms. The most common appears to be sensitivity to foods made with wheat flour. Other foods that could aggravate IBS include corn, eggs, soy, and highly processed snack foods. Eliminating them could help treat and prevent IBS. This has nothing to do with this subject, but nowadays I do try to eat only fresh food and avoid processed food. This is more to do with energy levels for me and nothing to do with my intestines.

If you want to try a systematic elimination diet, you should work with a clinical nutritionist, a registered dietitian, or a naturopath. Professionally supervised elimination diets vary, but most involve a week or two of eating a very restricted diet, followed by the reintroduction of foods one at a time. I did this, but without any results. If a newly reintroduced food provokes symptoms, that food is re-eliminated for a week or so, and then re-introduced. If it provokes symptoms again, you can feel confident that you're sensitive to it and eat it infrequently or not at all. An elimination diet might also help prevent IBS. Again, it's a case of listening to your body more than anything else.

- **Alkalizing**. As suggested before, for increased vitality and energy, it's worth pursuing a more "Alkaline" lifestyle. Many conditions are either caused by or exacerbated by too much acidity in the system, and the body does perform better in a slightly alkaline environment. So, it makes sense to do more in this way and generally become a bit healthier all round. For more information, just go to www.yourgutfeeling.com/energise.

Relaxation Therapies

Many studies have tested the effectiveness of relaxation therapies as a treatment. The various therapies—visualization, hypnotherapy, progressive muscle relaxation, biofeedback, meditation, and exercise—have consistently been shown to help. These methods, however, should not be viewed as separate. My treatment was a particular breed of hypnotherapy, combined with other relaxation techniques, such as visualization, muscle relaxation, learning to how to think, etc. These techniques were all entwined in Geoffrey's holistic methodology, which is perhaps why it is so powerful. I hope you're now confident of its safety and appropriateness for IBD problems.

- **Hypnotherapy**. With hypnotherapy, the hypnotherapist helps you become deeply relaxed using controlled breathing, powerful language techniques, muscle relaxation, guided imagery, and possibly music or a metronome. Once you're relaxed, you are more open to the positive guidance and suggestions that the therapist will put to you. This will help you visualize the result you want to achieve. Imagining this with great vividness will help direct your mind to achieving that goal. Read through my experiences with this earlier in this book where I tell you exactly how I used specific imagery and visualization to propel myself to complete fitness. Remember the fire engines putting out the fires in my body. Go back and look at Geoffrey's induction and my accompanying notes.

  Now, here's something interesting. Researchers in Bristol, England, treated thirty-three people with IBS with four forty-minute hypnotherapy sessions over seven weeks. At the end of the trial, eleven reported substantial reduction in their symptoms, and another nine reported improvement. In another study, fifty people whose IBS was poorly controlled by mainstream medications learned to relax deeply using hypnotherapy. Almost all of them (95 percent) experienced improvement, and when the researchers contacted them eighteen months later, those who continued their exercises reported lasting benefits. This is compelling evidence. Please pay it the respect it deserves. There is no other treatment I'm aware of with this high success rate.

- **Visualization**. Visualization is combined with the deep, meditative breathing and relaxation session. Imagining something like a beautiful scenario like a beach or a sunset in a panoramic meadow can help produce a calm feeling. The key to achieving deep relaxation through visualization is the content and vividness of the imagery. You don't just passively see a beach in your mind. You experience the rhythm of the waves, the warm glow of the sun, the softness of sand between your toes, and the ebb and flow of the tides.

- **Muscle relaxation**. It is thought that learning to relax your abdominal muscles can help symptoms of IBS. For me, I'd say that learning to relax *all* your muscles will be of help. Obviously, these will include your abdominal muscles, and this is part of the hypnotic induction outlined earlier in this course. Researchers at the Center for Stress and Anxiety Disorders at the State University of New York at Albany taught nineteen people with IBS a combination of progressive muscle relaxation (PMR) and biofeedback. PMR involves consciously relaxing one muscle group at a time until your whole body feels relaxed. Biofeedback is done through wiring certain muscle groups to a visual meter that displays their tension level. After PMR and biofeedback training, all the participants reported substantial improvement in IBS symptoms. Four years later, seventeen of the nineteen said they were still improved. If you listen and look at Geoffrey's hypnotic induction, you'll see that it does include muscle relaxation in groups. I adopt the same practice in my recording too.

- **Meditation**. Meditation involves sitting quietly with eyes closed, consciously emptying your mind, and focusing on a word or phrase (known as a mantra) or your breathing. The technique is usually practiced for about twenty minutes or longer once or twice a day. When thoughts come into your mind, you notice them, accept them, don't judge them, and then gently return to your mantra or breath.

A state of deep relaxation can contribute greatly to your health. It usually takes a month or two of daily practice before you begin to notice an enhanced feeling of general well-being. At the University Hospital of Wales in Cardiff, researchers studied thirty-five men and women with IBS. Some were given antispasmodic drugs, while others were enrolled in a stress management program involving meditation. Few of those in the drug group reported lasting improvement, but two-thirds of those practicing meditation did. A year later, most of the stress management group continued to report benefit.

- **Exercise**. This also has a calming effect. It releases endorphins, the body's own mood-elevating compounds. Most people who exercise regularly notice relaxation, an improved ability to cope with stress, and an enhanced feeling of general well-being. Naturopaths often recommend daily, leisurely twenty-minute walks for people with IBS.

- **Supplements**. It is thought that people with IBS may have unusually low levels of health-promoting ("probiotic") bacteria in their colons. Naturopaths suggest supplemental *Lactobacillus acidophilus* bacteria. *Acidophilus* supplements are commonly available nowadays and are popular with all sorts of people. Live culture yoghurt also contains *Acidophilus*, so there's another source.

- **Herbal medicine**. As discussed before, by all means experiment with herbal treatments. Provided you're sensible and do your research, they are unlikely to do any harm. Research has shown that traditional digestive herbs can be antispasmodic, meaning they relax the muscles surrounding the digestive tract. This helps prevent spasms that cause cramps and urgency.
  Several alcoholic drinks are herbal based and are thought to

have great benefits to the intestinal tract. These herbal drinks include Underberg, Jagermeister, and Ferna Branca. My favorite is Underberg, and I certainly will have a swig after a particularly over-excessive dinner, though I'm not recommending it as a medicine per se.

At the University of Exeter in England, researchers analyzed eight trials in which IBS was treated with peppermint oil. The results were positive, with subjects reporting that peppermint oil could be effective in providing some relief of IBS symptoms. Peppermint tea is also very calming and soothing, but research suggests it is absorbed into the bloodstream before it reaches the colon. Enteric-coated capsules of peppermint oil can get all the way to the colon before the coating dissolves and the oil is released. Enteric-coated peppermint oil capsules are available at many health food stores. As always, make sure you conduct proper research and follow the directions on the label ... and listen to your body.

- **Chinese medicine**. Apart from typically being absolutely disgusting to the taste, the main thing to watch for here is that your Chinese medicine practitioner knows what he or she is doing. The only real way to know this is by referral by someone who's had positive results from that practitioner. Chinese herb formulas for IBS vary, but they often include ginger root, ginseng root, licorice root, cinnamon twig, peony root, bupleurum root, and several other herbs that will insult your palate!

- **Acupuncture**. Chinese practitioners may also recommend acupuncture. I always found acupuncture very relaxing, so much so that it would always send me to sleep. This is a good start, but the other therapeutic factors need to be in place as well. Perhaps the ideal combination would be acupuncture combined with the hypnosis!

- **Homeopathy**. Homeopathy uses tiny microdoses of herbs and other substances to treat illness. It is very controversial. It didn't work for me, though some studies show that it can help treat a variety of conditions, including IBS. Personally, I have my doubts and have never met a homeopath who was truly convincing.

Colitis/Ulcerative Colitis

Ulcerative colitis is an inflammatory disease of the bowel that usually affects the distal end of the large intestine and rectum. The medical profession professes it to have no known cause, also stating there is a genetic component to susceptibility. Personally, I don't go along with either of these concepts, certainly not with my experience.

Symptoms

Chronic cases enduring over six months typically include diarrhea, which can be bloody and with no infective cause.

Inflammatory changes are most often confined to the left side and distal parts of the large intestine. However, any part of the colon can be affected. Inflammatory changes can expand over time and affect larger areas of the colon.

The disease can vary in severity from patient to patient and from time to time. It is thought that colitis is often found in former smokers (not me—I've never been a smoker). The theory goes that smoking can cause a reduction in the protective mucus lining the colon. When this protective mucus is reduced, the bacteria in the colon can attack the colon lining causing the immune system to become active and fight the bacteria. For unknown reasons, this causes damage to the lining (ulcers) of the colon walls in one or more places. Again, I am hugely skeptical about this theory.

Comparison to Crohn's Disease

Ulcerative colitis is similar to Crohn's disease, but there are characteristic differences. Ulcerative colitis affects only the colon and does not "migrate" to the small intestine, while Crohn's disease can affect the entire digestive tract. It is usually confined to the mucosal and submucosal lining of the colon, and affects whole areas of intestine. Crohn's disease, on the other hand, tends to be patchy and affect more layers of intestine, being transmural in nature. Due to the nature of the inflammation, ulcerative colitis is rarely considered for resection surgery, in contrast to Crohn's disease, where such surgery is often used due to dangerous bowel obstructions and other complications.

Diagnosis and Prognosis

Continuous bloody diarrhea (the severity of which is variable from time to time), with no sign of infection or fever, is consistent with ulcerative colitis. A diagnosis is usually achieved through colonoscopy (up periscope!) with biopsy of pathological lesions. Ulcerative colitis most often affects the rectum and the distal left side of the colon, but can occur anywhere in the large intestine.

In many ulcerative colitis cases, prognosis can be relatively good, as symptom relief can often be maintained through relatively harmless anti-inflammatory medication, and most patients may never require any kind of surgery for their condition. While quality of life can often be impaired by unpleasant symptoms such as pain and chronic diarrhea, the disease is very rarely fatal on its own, and many patients enjoy normal symptom-free lives while in remission.

Treatment

Although some progress has been made in the last twenty years in understanding and treating the disease, a definitive treatment or cure for ulcerative colitis still eludes modern medicine. Therefore, conventional treatment for ulcerative colitis actually aims at inducing remission, preventing relapse, improving nutritional deficiency, and in child patients, ensuring normal growth and development.

Anti-inflammatory drugs (such as sulfasalazine or mesalazine) are often used, and in severe cases, corticosteroids may be given. Immunosuppressive agents such as azathioprine, 6-mercaptopurine (6-MP), and more recently, cyclosporine are also used as preventive medications. Anti-diarrheal drugs (such as loperamide) should only be used under specific doctors' orders, as they can aggravate the condition.

Surgery is rarely recommended to treat ulcerative colitis except in cases where drug treatment has proven completely ineffective and where the condition is acute. (Remember, that was my position in April 1995). Since ulcerative colitis affects only the colon, a complete large intestine removal is considered to be a cure of sorts by the medical profession (albeit highly unsatisfactory). However, this option would leave the patient with a permanent ileostomy, which can cause further problems in itself, not to mention the adverse psychological effect. A more aesthetically and functionally pleasing resolution may be a j-pouch surgery, where a part of the terminal ileum is used to create a "pouch," which is then connected to the anus. This preserves the appearance of normal bowel function, although bowel movements are somewhat more frequent.

There is no proven connection between dietary habits and the onset of the disease. Although opinions are somewhat divided on this issue, it is reasonable to say that no particular diet can influence length of remission or cause inflammation if none is present; this is certainly consistent with my experience. The usual recommendation for patients is to simply avoid foods that have caused them discomfort in the past, and try to eat as healthy as possible for overall nutritional value.

Ongoing Research

The medical profession states that definitive cause of ulcerative colitis may never be discovered, since it is highly possible that it is a result of a combination of environmental, genetic, bacterial, and other factors. Nevertheless, they state that an effective treatment or even a cure may not be very far away. That would be great. Whatever works is all that matters. There is much research currently being conducted in this area, with some new theories and medications that are said to be showing promising results. However, during the last nine years that I have been well, I haven't seen nearly as much in the way of progress in this area that I would have expected all that time ago. Some open-mindedness as to the cause would, I believe, be helpful.

Recently, probiotics have become a powerful alternative treatment for ulcerative colitis. While they do not cure the disease, they have been found to significantly reduce symptoms. One probiotic formula known as VSL #3 is said to have shown promise for people with ulcerative colitis.

Crohn's Disease

Definition

A chronic form of inflammatory bowel disease, Crohn's disease causes severe irritation in the gastrointestinal tract. It usually affects the lower small intestine (called the ileum) or the colon, but is different from colitis in that it can affect the entire gastrointestinal tract.

About 30 percent of all Crohn's disease cases involve only the small bowel. About half of all cases involve the small bowel and colon and about 20 percent of all cases affect the colon alone.

Causes and Risk Factors of Crohn's Disease

For my money there are too many common denominators between Crohn's, colitis, and IBS; however, the cause of Crohn's disease is defined as unknown by the medical profession. They still suggest that genetics, infection, altered immunity, and psychological factors may all play a role. I believe the psychological factors should be investigated more thoroughly.

The disease is thought to have a peak occurrence between the ages of fifteen and thirty-five, though it has been reported in every decade of life. The condition is more common in Caucasians, and it can affect more than one member of a family. While some researchers believe (wrongly in my opinion) that viruses and bacteria can cause colitis, little evidence suggests that infections actually lead to Crohn's disease. For my money, I think that little evidence suggests likewise for colitis.

Symptoms of Crohn's Disease

Because of the varying locations of involvement and severity of disease, Crohn's disease may present with a variety of symptoms and signs. The first symptoms of Crohn's disease are often abdominal pain and diarrhea. Pain is felt in the area of the navel or on the right side and often follows a meal. Pain in the joints, lack of appetite, weight loss, and fever are also common. This makes common sense because, as I mentioned before, feeling bloated and uncomfortable in the stomach hardly lends itself to a large appetite.

Diagnosis

There is a poor correlation between laboratory studies and the patient's clinical picture. Laboratory values may reflect inflammatory activity or the nutritional effects of the disease. Often, radiological tests include an upper gastrointestinal series with a small bowel follow-through study to look for ulcerations or fistulas. To evaluate the colon, a colonoscopy or barium enema may be performed.

Treatment

Since no specific therapy exists, current clinical treatment targets symptomatic improvement and control of the disease process. I find this attitude to the condition very narrow minded. Dietary restrictions vary from patient to patient, but there is no definitive evidence of a specific food allergy causing the disease.

The cornerstone of clinical treatment for acute and severe Crohn's disease continues to be corticosteroids. They also have a role in managing less severe disease and in treating small bowel involvement. They are used for short-term therapy. Anti-diarrhea drugs can improve the quality of life. The risk of adverse effects from opioid agents, such as loperamide HCL, is low if the patient does not have active severe colitis. A high percentage of patients will respond to a course of prednisone, although the endoscopic appearance may remain unchanged, meaning the disease hasn't gone. Corticosteroids plus sulfasalazine may yield an encouraging initial result, but the overall outcome is likely to be the same.

Antibiotic agents, such as metronidazole (Flagyl and Protostat), may be helpful in perineal Crohn's disease. The drug must be used with caution, however, because the therapeutic window is small, and effective doses may cause peripheral nervous system toxicity.

Immunosuppressive drugs can be effective in treating Crohn's disease. However, despite advances in the medical treatment of Crohn's, surgery may still be advised in order to remove the diseased segment of bowel. Surgery is usually suggested for those whom medical treatment has been ineffective. Remember, that's what I was recommended in April 1995. It's difficult for me to make comment on for individual cases. All I can keep doing is reminding people that surgery was proposed for me and I emphatically rejected it. There are other occasions where surgery may be advised. These include:

- permanent narrowing or an obstruction of the bowel
- development of a fistula between an involved segment and the bladder, vagina, or skin
- infection in the area of the anus
- perforation of the bowel
- abscess (localized infection) within the abdomen
- extreme widening (toxic dilation) of the colon

Here's the real kick in the teeth: Crohn's disease can recur after surgery, even if the surgeon removes all traces of the disease. The same applies with colitis. And that's one of the many reasons I turned down surgery. However, despite the serious nature of the disease, treatment often permits the person with Crohn's disease to lead an active and productive life. In my case, the colitis was horrendously painful and was accompanied by virtual incontinence, so there was very little quality of life. This may have been one of the many reasons that led to my determination to seek other methods of treatment.

BUY A SHARE OF THE FUTURE IN YOUR COMMUNITY

These certificates make great holiday, graduation and birthday gifts that can be personalized with the recipient's name. The cost of one S.H.A.R.E. or one square foot is $54.17. The personalized certificate is suitable for framing and will state the number of shares purchased and the amount of each share, as well as the recipient's name. The home that you participate in "building" will last for many years and will continue to grow in value.

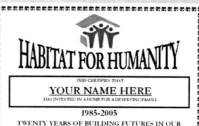

Here is a sample SHARE certificate:

HABITAT FOR HUMANITY

THIS CERTIFIES THAT
YOUR NAME HERE
HAS INVESTED IN A HOME FOR A DESERVING FAMILY

1985-2005
TWENTY YEARS OF BUILDING FUTURES IN OUR
COMMUNITY ONE HOME AT A TIME

1200 SQUARE FOOT HOUSE @ $65,000 = $54.17 PER SQUARE FOOT
This certificate represents a tax deductible donation. It has no cash value.

YES, I WOULD LIKE TO HELP!

I support the work that Habitat for Humanity does and I want to be part of the excitement! As a donor, I will receive periodic updates on your construction activities but, more importantly, I know my gift will help a family in our community realize the dream of homeownership. **I would like to SHARE in your efforts against substandard housing in my community!** *(Please print below)*

PLEASE SEND ME _____ SHARES at $54.17 EACH = $ $_____

In Honor Of: _____

Occasion: (Circle One)   *HOLIDAY*   *BIRTHDAY*   *ANNIVERSARY*

     OTHER: _____

Address of Recipient: _____

Gift From: _____ *Donor Address:* _____

Donor Email: _____

I AM ENCLOSING A CHECK FOR $ $_____ PAYABLE TO HABITAT FOR HUMANITY <u>OR</u> PLEASE CHARGE MY VISA OR MASTERCARD *(CIRCLE ONE)*

Card Number _____ Expiration Date: _____

Name as it appears on Credit Card _____ Charge Amount $ _____

Signature _____

Billing Address _____

Telephone # Day _____ Eve _____

PLEASE NOTE: Your contribution is tax-deductible to the fullest extent allowed by law.
Habitat for Humanity • P.O. Box 1443 • Newport News, VA 23601 • 757-596-5553
www.HelpHabitatforHumanity.org

LaVergne, TN USA
08 April 2010
178618LV00004B/91/P